WIDE AWAKE

AND

DREAMING

A MEMOIR OF NARCOLEPSY

Julie Flygare

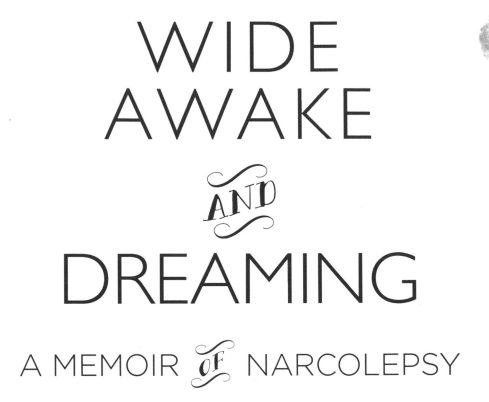

PRAISE *for*
WIDE AWAKE AND DREAMING

" If you want to find out what it is like to have narcolepsy, you must read *Wide Awake and Dreaming*. Julie's memoir is so well written with such interesting and entertaining detail, honesty and openness. Julie describes her story so clearly as 'her' story and yet, many people will recognize their own story in here. A wonderful recommended must read for everyone! Julie is a natural story teller."

-EVELINE HONIG, M.D., M.P.H.

Executive Director, Narcolepsy Network, Inc.

" A tender and compelling tale of a young woman's frightening journey, attempting to make sense of medical symptoms associated with a disorder of which few physicians are aware or comprehend. It is a search for both internal understanding and a quest for diagnosis and treatment of this sleep-related disorder that afflicts many unsuspecting women and men. It is a sensitive plea to health care providers to become aware of narcolepsy and cataplexy so early diagnosis and management can be instituted in order to avoid the intense impact of delayed diagnosis."

-STEPHEN H. SHELDON, D.O., F.A.A.P.

Director, Sleep Medicine Center, Ann and Robert H. Lurie Children's Hospital of Chicago

Professor of Pediatrics, Northwestern University Feinberg School of Medicine

"Julie shares her story brilliantly. She relates the details in such a way, that it is an easy read with snippets of humor added. This, I believe, makes her an ideal spokesperson for narcolepsy. Julie is all about helping others to empower themselves; to make their journey into the unknown a little less scary than it was for her. She uses her own life's experiences to teach us how to find humor, and hope, in our own health circumstances. Whether you have narcolepsy, or another condition, this is a must read book."
-MICHELLE KING ROBSON
Founder and Chairperson, EmpowHER

"Narcolepsy is so often misunderstood and patients frequently feel alone. Julie's memoir is a relatable, comforting account that everyone with narcolepsy or who knows someone with narcolepsy should read."
-MALI EINEN
PWN and Clinical Coordinator, Stanford University Center for Narcolepsy

"Thoughtfully written, *Wide Awake and Dreaming* offers a brave and honest account of one woman's struggle with narcolepsy. This eloquent memoir will provide solace, hope and strength to others dealing with such a highly misunderstood and stigmatized disorder."
-SHELBY FREEDMAN HARRIS, PSY.D., C.BSM
Director of the Behavioral Sleep Medicine Program, Montefiore Medical Center's Sleep-Wake Disorders Center
Assistant Professor of Neurology and Psychiatry, Albert Einstein College of Medicine

PRAISE *for*
JULIE FLYGARE'S BLOG

" Julie Flygare tends to not let little things like impossibilities get in her way. Her positive attitude and genuine writings about who she is and how she deals with her disorder will take her further than she could ever hope to run. She is easily one of the more inspirational people I have met." **–M.C.**

" I so admire how you took this trial and grew from it and allowed good to come of it. I am grateful for your strong, articulate voice and your willingness to share your story. So thank you for opening up and allowing others to learn and grow along with you." -L.W.

" Thank you for caring, thank you for dedicating your life, when you could have just went on and been a great lawyer. Thank you for giving narcolepsy a face. Thank you for making a difference for all of us struggling." **-S.B.**

" I've had narcolepsy for twelve years now and for practically all of it, I would have rather buried it in order to appear more normal, but seeing the way that you deal with it and let others know about it has really inspired me to be more accepting of it. Thanks for showing me a better way of dealing with this thing that is narcolepsy." **-C.S.**

" You are part of the inspiration that has driven me to get better and try new, or old, things that I have wanted to do, or did in the past." -**C.G.**

" I am amazed at your talent to communicate and get narcolepsy out there. You are an inspiration! Keep it up." -**K.H.**

" I find myself returning to your blog for continued inspiration and help with changing my outlook on life. You've shown me how accepting the diagnosis does not mean that my life must be less full." -**A.C.**

" Your dedication is inspiring. Using this blog to make others aware of narcolepsy and sleep disorders is truly wonderful. Because narcolepsy has no cure, it becomes a management issue. We are cheering for you from Maryland!" -**S.K.**

" The worst thing we can do to someone is to take away hope. Thank you, Julie, for giving and keeping alive, the hope that life can and will get better for those afflicted with narcolepsy." -**M.L.**

WIDE AWAKE

AND

DREAMING

A MEMOIR OF NARCOLEPSY

Julie Flygare

WIDE AWAKE AND DREAMING
A Memoir of Narcolepsy

AUTHOR'S NOTE:
The names and other identifying details of some major and minor characters have been changed to protect individual privacy and anonymity.

PUBLISHER:
Mill Pond Swan Publishing
Arlington, VA

ISBN: 978-0-9883149-0-0

LIBRARY OF CONGRESS CONTROL NUMBER: 2012922451

BOOK COVER:
Cover Design: Cecilia Sorochin
Cover Art: Lucy Hillenbrand
Photo: Matthew Spaulding

Interior Design: Cecilia Sorochin

Quantity discounts are available for educational or business uses. For more information, please contact Mill Pond Swan Publishing, PO Box 3543, Arlington, VA 22203 or millpondswan@gmail.com.

www.julieflygare.com

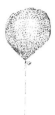

In loving memory,

THOMAS JOHN FLYGARE

"And if our hands should meet in another dream,
we shall build another tower in the sky."

-KAHLIL GIBRAN

CONTENTS

"WAKE BUTTERFLY, IT'S LATE
AND WE'VE MILES TO GO TOGETHER."

-Basho

ONE
MELTING

I T BEGAN WITH LAUGHTER.

Deep mustard-colored beams of late afternoon light spread across the hardwood floors. The scents of fresh mulch and thawing mud sifted in through the open bay windows at the front of the room. An unseasonably warm spring breeze whispered in my ear, "You should really be outside."

It was the spring of 2006 and I was looking forward to my run along the Charles River, knowing it was one of those perfect days that would remind me just how much I loved Boston.

After graduating from Brown University in 2005, I'd moved into my first grown-up apartment with a good friend, Jill, in the picturesque Fenway neighborhood of Boston. Working as a file clerk at a fancy law firm was, thankfully, a limited time engagement since I was recently admitted to law school. Jill taught kindergarten and her misadventures were a constant source of entertainment in our apartment – a breath of fresh air in our budding adult lives.

"He asked for Cheerios, so I gave him Cheerios."

"Wait, isn't this the same boy that stuck Cheerios up his nose last week?" I asked.

"Well yes, but – "

"Jill, you shouldn't have given him Cheerios again. "

"I know! But I was distracted."

Sensing where this was going, I chuckled to myself as I crouched down to double-knot my sneakers. I was wearing a baggy white t-shirt and my favorite mint green running shorts; my iPod was on the kitchen counter, charged and ready to go. I stood tall and sturdy, supported by my cushioned Asics and muscular legs.

"No longer than *ten* seconds later," Jill continued, "I heard snickers behind me."

"Oh *no*, not again."

"Oh *yes*, and worse than last time! His nostrils were flared like an angry bull, chock-full of Cheerios!"

Jill raised both pointer fingers and tugged grotesquely at her nostrils. We burst out laughing. Poor Jill, never a dull moment. I imagined the little half-boy, half-bull, smiling ear to ear.

Then, in the midst of laughter, my knees melted, as if someone had poked behind them, breaking their locked stance momentarily.

"Did you see that?"

"See what?" Jill's eyes were still sparkling with humor.

"My knees, they just did the strangest thing – gave out on me, sort of."

Of course Jill hadn't noticed anything. It happened so quickly, as if I'd fallen, but only on the inside, while remaining steady on the outside. How odd, I thought.

I walked around the apartment for a few minutes, testing my legs for signs of weakness. Everything seemed normal, so I grabbed my iPod and left for my run as planned.

Outdoors, my hesitation quickly faded, as my knees caught each stride with power and ease. Running was mindless – my escape from life's stresses.

As a young girl growing up in a small town in New Hampshire, I had looked upon Boston with wide eyes when my mother drove my sister, Michelle, my brother, Travis and me to see the Egyptian mummies and Impressionist paintings at the Museum of Fine Arts. On special occasions, Mom took us for homemade cannolis in the North End, the Italian section of Boston. Usually, Mom was very health conscious, standing only five feet tall she watched her diet and exercised regularly, but cannolis were her weakness. We loaded up on powdered sugar and took ravenous bites of the vanilla and ricotta cheese filled pastries.

While attending high school 20 minutes outside the city, I had often lingered in front of expensive boutiques on Newbury Street, staring at the mannequins and daydreaming about wearing those same silk fabrics. As a student at Brown University in nearby Providence, I had spent every summer living in Boston – teaching tennis at Harvard and running along the Charles River.

Now, at age 22, my favorite view of the city was on my running path, just after crossing the Boston University Bridge. It was here that I caught all of Boston in a single glance – from the lights of Fenway Park to the brilliant gold dome of the State House, the sleek Hancock building and boxy Prudential tower.

As I ran along the Charles River on this beautiful spring day, I breathed deeply to take it all in. The path was already very familiar and now, with my recent acceptance to Boston College Law School, I'd continue running this same route for many more years to come. My appetite for Boston was insatiable. The streets, the buildings, the restaurants, the Red Sox, the running paths – all carried me.

Outside my apartment building, I walked with my hands on my head to catch my breath. The wet neckline of my t-shirt suctioned against my hot chest. As the daylight faded, I leaned against a cement column to stretch my calves and quads – bending and straightening my limbs like Play-Doh.

By nightfall, I dismissed the strange knee melting that had come out of nowhere. It was gone before I was sure of its existence.

A month later, I stood talking with a group of friends at a dinner party. Someone said something funny and as I laughed, my knees slid out from under me for a split second. I looked at my lower body, wondering what had just happened.

My friends continued joking. The weakness passed so quickly, I assumed they didn't notice, but the first incident from the month before came back like déjà vu. Although I'd been laughing both times, I wasn't sure laughter was to blame, until my knees buckled a third time, again while I was standing and laughing.

Over the summer, "my knee thing" returned every couple of weeks, always when I was laughing, though not every time I laughed. I tried to control my laughter, but despite my best efforts, laughter still managed to slip into my days, to enliven my spirit, and simultaneously weaken my knees.

At work, the monotony of my job bored me, so I visited my friend Elise's cubicle to break things up. Both file clerks en route to law school, we enjoyed each other's company so much that our conversations often led to laughter and my knee thing.

I sensed that when a wave-like fog came over me as I laughed, I was on the verge of losing my knees. Elise and I were having a funny conversation one day, and when my head started to tingle, I knew the fog was coming.

"Elise, don't make me laugh! My knee thing…"

It was no use, the progression from laughter to weakness was too quick. I reached for her desk to brace myself, knowing that I could count on a solid object to support me when my own legs couldn't.

Although I had described to Elise how my knees buckled when things were funny, she never noticed any jerking or strange motions in my legs. She only saw me move toward the desk for support. I began to wonder if I was really on the verge of falling or if I just *thought* I was falling. It felt very physical, yet I couldn't be sure, because the incidents remained invisible to those around me. I asked friends and family members if they'd heard of anything like this before, but they only responded with blank stares.

M id-summer 2006, I realized I needed a doctor to sign off on my health for law school – just a standard physical and official proof of my vaccination history. No problem, except that I didn't have a doctor.

I'd gone to a pediatrician until the age of 18 and while in college, I had used the health services on campus. In the year since graduating, I hadn't needed a doctor. Now, I needed someone to say I was healthy, and quickly. There was threatening language about what would happen if my forms weren't in on time, so Mom made an appointment for me at an OB-GYN office in New Hampshire where one of her tennis friends worked. I loathed doctor's offices, so I was happy to let Mom coordinate the transfer of my medical records from my pediatrician's office to the OBGYN.

On the day of my appointment, a nurse greeted me in the OBGYN's waiting room and led the way to an examination room, where a light green smock lay neatly folded on the examination table.

Once alone, I undressed to my underwear and lifted the smock up in the air – trying to remember how to wear it. I finally wrapped the thin cloth around my body and climbed onto the table. The protective paper crinkled under my thighs. The hair on my arms stood up straight. Thick frosty air poured in from the air conditioner, making me shiver.

Soon, the doctor knocked and came in to begin her examination. She was friendly and efficient. Good this, great that, perfect here, looks fine there.

"So, are you excited for law school?"

"Oh yes, very excited, but also nervous." This was the truth. I had mixed feelings.

She smiled and held out my paperwork, "Good luck. I'm sure you'll do great."

I took the papers – all the proper boxes were checked and she had signed and dated everything accordingly. I'd been so focused on finalizing the forms for law school, I forgot to ask about my knee thing until the doctor turned to leave.

"Wait, there's one thing I was curious about."

She swung back around, her arms hugged around my closed file.

"Sometimes when I'm laughing, my knees give out on me. They break their locked stance and regain strength quickly, as if someone poked behind them unexpectedly."

"Only when you're laughing?"

"Yes, not every time, but sometimes, my laughter is accompanied by a slight tingling in my head and then my knees buckle."

"Try breathing deeper when you laugh."

Try breathing deeper? I didn't think breathing had anything to do with my knee thing, but she seemed sure of her advice, and who was I to tell her she was wrong?

As she ducked out the door, I thanked her and started putting my clothes back on. She must have thought I was laughing too hard and not getting enough oxygen; on the verge of fainting perhaps. If only I could start over and explain it again, surely she'd know what I was talking about and come up with a solution.

Once dressed, I grabbed my paperwork and flung the door open, leaving the frigid twilight zone of medicine and heading back into the sultry August sunshine. I sped off to the post office to mail the forms – hoping my perfect health report would arrive in time. After the appointment, I never tried breathing deeper when I laughed because I knew it wouldn't help. Although my knee issue worried me, law school was my most pressing concern.

TWO
LIGHTS OUT

E AST WING 115 WAS a newly remodeled stadium-style classroom in
the basement of Boston College Law School, where my Property
Law class was held. Instead of windows, only a few orange-tinted
bulbs dimly lit the subterranean room. Silhouettes filed in from the hallway. The projector hummed softly, emanating a stream of blue and green
flickers onto the large screen at the front of the room.

Everything was state-of-the-art; from the wireless internet and electrical outlets at each seat to the rotating chalkboards, dry erase boards and
projection screens. My law school section, all 85 of us, settled along the
various tiers of the underground coliseum, staring into glowing laptop
screens – our only connection to the outside world.

At the front of the room, a quiet man in his 40s, Professor Liu, stood
looking into his own computer screen, preparing to start our class. A few
students chatted softly with neighbors. I fanned through the 1,000-page
textbook to find the cases assigned for the day.

At exactly 2 p.m., Professor Liu looked out at the students and everyone fell silent. He opened his mouth to inhale, and we placed our hands above our keyboards as if he was the conductor of a grand orchestra.

When he spoke, the clicking began, softly at first, in the front row with the especially eager students typing away. As he continued on past logistic announcements into course material, more students joined in the chorus, reaching a crescendo about 20 minutes into class, when Professor Liu made a particularly important point. At that time, the entire room fluttered with the pitter-patter of various electronic notes.

At this point, we were only a few weeks into our first semester and our note-taking was mostly word-for-word lecture transcription. I was still learning to interpret the language of the law, so I followed along, typing almost every word that crossed Professor Liu's lips, afraid I might miss a nugget of wisdom that would be on the exam – the key point that would be the difference between an A and a B, the divide between getting the big, fancy job I wanted and being rejected.

Yet, this particular day my desire to record every second of class came up against another, equally strong desire – a dark and unwelcome compulsion to go to sleep.

About half way through the class, a heaviness came over my head, with a weight sitting on my skull. Next, my shoulders and elbows began to ache and a wave of nausea crawled up my stomach. I shifted in my chair to find a more comfortable position and stretched my head to one side and then the other, hoping to dislodge the uneasiness swelling inside me.

Property class was an hour and 20 minutes long. I checked the clock on my computer; it was 2:52 p.m. – only 28 more minutes to go. I returned to typing feverishly.

I tried to ignore the burning sensation at the back of my eyes but the harder I worked to keep my eyelids open, the more it felt like a ferocious fire blazing behind them. I glanced at the bottom of my computer, 2:53 p.m.

Soon, Professor Liu's voice faded. Some of his words echoed over and over while others went missing. I squinted to try to read the large font of his slideshow. My typing slowed to a lethargic pace. The lecture slipped like sand through my fingers.

Eyes open, Julie. Just keep your – –

Next, I opened my eyes and made direct eye contact with Professor Liu. I had no idea how long my eyes had been closed. Embarrassment flooded my body, and suddenly, I was freed from my struggle against sleep. The weight lifted off my skull and the flames died down behind my eyes.

All too soon, the heaviness returned and began seeping downward in my skull, sucking at my strength again. The time was now 3:03 p.m. I walked out into the hallway. Dizzy and only partially aware of my sur-roundings, I wandered toward the bathroom, as if through a fun-house wavy mirror maze.

I stumbled into a stall and sat down. My head collapsed over my arms and legs. I just needed to rest. Consciousness drifted from me and I started sliding off the toilet seat. I whipped back to attention. The bathroom was silent. Thankfully no one else was there.

The heaviness still sat on my skull. My mind teetered between the bath-room and darkness. I tried pinching the skin of my forearms to wake up. I started slapping my face. With increasing intensity, I slapped myself again and again as hard as possible. These slaps were satisfying, not only because they woke me up, but also because they released a rage in me for not hav-ing the backbone and discipline to perform the simplest of tasks, of *just… staying… awake.* When I'd had enough, I jumped up and down a few times, like a boxer preparing to enter the ring.

Out of the stall, I looked in the mirror at the girl with glassed-over eyes. *What is your problem?* I splashed cold water on my face and patted a wet paper towel under my chin and against the back of my neck, hoping to refresh myself.

I took a few deep breaths and re-arranged my hair to curve my bangs over my forehead. I straightened the collar of my pink dress shirt. On the outside, everything looked right.

The fog had lifted. I returned to class with eyes turned downward, hoping Professor Liu wouldn't notice me again, the same student who he'd caught sleeping minutes earlier. The time was 3:13 p.m. I'd missed 10 minutes of precious lecture time.

Placing my hands back on my keyboard, I scrolled up to review my notes. The top of the page was organized neatly in a variety of fonts and bullet points. Half way down, the order fell to pieces – with half-sentences, words standing alone, and even letters that formed no words at all. Legal terms co-mingled with random places and names from outside of law school. My stomach tightened. I'd interwoven the lecture with a dream in a nonsensical stream of consciousness.

Drawing my cursor over the scrambled words, I quickly erased the gibberish.

The last few minutes of class passed fairly smoothly, with only a few minor dips toward sleepiness. I closed down my computer after class, knowing there were major gaps in my notes, but I'd have to catch up later. What concerned me most was escaping the law school basement.

Within minutes, I flung open the heavy metal door to the parking lot. A crisp breeze greeted me, cutting across my face. I leaned my head back and smiled. The fresh air was invigorating. Delicate hints of yellow and orange laced the tree leaves overhead. Autumn was on its way.

By 5 p.m., I was on a treadmill at the gym, on track to go seven miles in an hour. My reflection bounced along in the full-length mirror – legs lunging forward, arms pumping and head bouncing in rhythm. My body and mind were one.

Some people had speculated that law school would keep me too busy to stay in shape, but I'd laughed at these predictions. I knew that much of my time in law school would be spent silently hunched over a computer or book and running would be more important than ever for balance. The weight in my skull never touched me in the gym. During my workouts, I was free.

Returning home, I showered, ate dinner and got ready to start my home-work. Sitting upright in bed, surrounded by textbooks, highlighters, and a laptop, I read the first paragraph of the first case assigned for my Contracts Law class. Within seconds, my brain shut down. There was no fighting, no fire in my eyes, no aching muscles – I went out quickly and smoothly, slumped over a night's worth of homework.

Around midnight, my consciousness re-surfaced and although I was ex-hausted, I brushed my teeth, set my alarm for 5 a.m., turned out the lights and went to sleep again.

It was still dark out when my alarm went off. Every bone in my body wanted to stay in bed, but I forced myself to go sit at the table in the cold living room and read my homework. My Contracts Professor used the "So-cratic Method" – cold-calling on students at random to answer questions in front of the entire class. If I hadn't done my homework and got called on, all 85 of my peers and my professor would know it.

I worked for three hours before getting dressed for school, but even this wasn't enough time to finish all my assigned reading for the day. I'd have to skim the rest quickly in the breaks between classes.

Although the school week was always a tough sprint to the finish, the weekends were much more enjoyable. Each Saturday morn-ing of the fall semester, I laced up my running sneakers, grabbed an old leather baseball mitt and drove a few miles to Cleveland Park in Brighton to join my section's softball team. All the first year sections fielded teams in the law school softball league and there were teams made up of second and third year students.

One Saturday, I arrived at the field as my team captain announced the line up.

"Julie, you're up third."

I scanned the dew-laden grass for my favorite bat. "Who are we playing?"

"They're second year students and by the looks of them, serious about softball."

A tall female player stood on the mound, stretching her pitching arm, as the all-male infielders aggressively hurled the softball around the diamond to warm up.

Growing up, softball was never my favorite sport, but as a trained squash and tennis player, my hand-eye coordination was decent and because I was a runner, I had good speed. The week before, I had gotten on base three out of four times at bat.

When it was my turn at bat, I sauntered to the plate, head held high. A few of my teammates cheered, "Okay, Julie, here we go!" and "Just like last week, Flygare."

I lifted the bat for the first pitch, when a deep male voice from the field yelled, "Easy out! Easy out!"

I lowered the bat slightly and glared toward first base. A male player leaned forward with his mitt open, as if about to catch a ball.

My teammates responded, "Booo!"

"You show him, Flygare," my captain chimed in.

I shifted my stance and refocused my attention on the female pitcher, as she launched the softball into the air. It arched up, and then fell low to the ground by my knees. I gripped the bat and swung with all my might.

Crack! The crisp sound of perfect contact rang across the field as the ball soared through the gap between first and second base. I dropped the bat and sprinted to first base, with plenty of time before the outfielder got the ball to the first baseman. I jumped up and down on the bag and pumped my fists overhead like an Olympic gold medalist. My teammates hooted and hollered from the bench, laughing at the first baseman who had mistaken me for a less advanced player.

"Nice hit." He threw the ball to the pitcher.

"Thanks!" I beamed inside and out.

When the first baseman came up to bat in the next inning, I couldn't help yelling, "Easy out!"

Everyone chuckled before he hammered the ball over our outfielders' heads for a triple. I made it a point to remember his name when one of his teammates called him Taylor.

The following Saturday, I was en route to meet up with my team when I noticed Taylor sitting on a nearby bench. As I passed by, he stood up.

"Hey there!"

"Hi." I smiled.

"Sorry about last week. I was trying to psych you out, but you proved me wrong!"

I giggled, "That's fine. It was a really fun game."

"I'm Taylor, by the way."

I reached out to shake his hand. "I'm Julie."

Taylor's tight t-shirt showed off his muscular shoulders and arms. He was tall, with a nice smile and shaggy brown hair. A typical sporty New England boy – rough around the edges with boyish facial features. As we continued talking, his gentle demeanor intrigued me as somehow in conflict with his macho appearance. We went our separate ways, but after that, I kept an eye out for him at school.

The day after Thanksgiving, I left my family early in the morning to return to campus. I carried my laptop in one arm and Property Law textbook in the other, to the top floor of the library and peered over the banister, hoping to see friendly faces or the cute softball player, Taylor. The spacious tables and numerous study carols, usually overflowing with students, were empty. Only one individual sat inside the third floor computer lab.

The stark vacancy of the library surprised me, since the end of the semester was quickly approaching and the first year students' Property Law exam was less than two weeks away. *My dedication must be stronger than my classmates*, I thought, as I waltzed down a deserted row of study carols.

Within a few hours, I peeled the right side of my face off the page of my textbook, only to find drool on the case I was supposed to be reading. My neck and shoulders were stiff from the awkward position. I wiped my spit off the page and returned to work.

Warm heat emanated from a nearby vent, softly purring in the stagnant airspace. I'd been trying to grasp the differences between Fee Simple Absolute, Fee Simple Determinable, Fee Simple Subject to a Condition Subsequent, and Fee Simple Subject to an Executory Limitation all morning, but my brain refused to cooperate. Outside, brown leaves fell from trees and whipped around in dusty spirals of whistling wind. Inside, the library remained tranquil – perhaps too tranquil.

In the few hours I'd been studying, I had taken two naps and barely made a dent in my workload. This extra day of studying could have given me an enormous advantage over my classmates, yet my Property Law textbook had been reduced to an uncomfortable pillow.

This wasn't my first encounter with tedious dry subject matters. As an art history major in college, I'd memorized the titles, artists and dates of hundreds of art works and scored high on the exams. Somehow, law school was challenging me in new ways.

Staring blankly at the text, I questioned whether I'd lost the discipline and will power to focus on intellectually challenging material. I closed the book, shut down my computer and left the library.

I had recognized the melting in my knees with laughter as new and unusual right away. The tiredness, however, crept in more slowly so I didn't realize it was getting worse. In the midst of a jam-packed schedule of academic, athletic and social commitments, my sleepiness stayed under the radar for quite a while.

There were plenty of logical excuses for my tiredness, I reasoned. Dark rooms were the problem. Hot rooms, too. I wasn't a morning person or a night owl. I was sleepy because I just ate, or worked out. I hadn't had enough caffeine, or I'd had too much. And so on.

Once, studying in my undergraduate college library, I was more tired than usual, but didn't give it much thought. My list of excuses then included intense practices with the varsity squash team, sometimes twice a day, and staying up late studying or socializing. There were so many legitimate reasons for sleepiness in college; I grew accustomed to the fog. By my junior year, I'd perfected the ritual of going to the bathroom during class to wake myself. I'd continued the same tactics in my first semester of law school.

One day in early January, I almost ran into Taylor while walking through a corridor at school. We hadn't crossed paths since softball last fall.

"You still go to this school?"

He chuckled and stopped to chat. Making small talk, we discovered that he'd gone to a college with a squash team that was a rival of mine.

"I'm pretty sure that my team beat yours most of the time." He smiled.

"Excuse me? Not in the years I was on the team." I couldn't remember if this was entirely true, but it didn't matter.

After bantering a few more minutes, I scurried along to class. Later that day, an email showed up in my school inbox from Taylor with an article about his school's squash team beating mine. My heart raced as I opened it.

For about a week, we exchanged emails until eventually, he asked if I'd like to grab a drink. Two nights later, in the bitter cold of January, we met at a local sports bar in my neighborhood and talked over a few beers. After my second drink, the warm fuzzy effects of the alcohol began to set in.

Taylor accompanied me home from the bar. Passing Fenway Park, a big gust of wind hit us front on. He pulled me toward him for warmth and I relaxed easily into the space between his arm and chest. The closeness felt right. At my doorstep, he kissed me goodnight and we made plans to see each other that weekend. Within a week, we'd been on three dates.

One evening not long after we started dating, I sat in the privacy of my bedroom and anxiously logged onto the school's online transcript program to check my first semester grades. B- in Property, B- in Torts and C+ in Contracts – the worst grades of my academic career. I sat in silence for a few minutes, absolutely stunned, until reality sank in and shock turned to devastation. Tears fell uncontrollably down my cheeks.

I called Taylor and asked him to come over. Although things were still new between us, when he heard the quiver in my voice, he agreed to come immediately.

He lived in Brighton, five miles away, but arrived within minutes. Trying to cheer me up, he reminded me that these were only three grades.

"You'll get another five in the spring. You can bounce back. It'll be okay."

I didn't know why he believed in me so much, but I hoped he was right. We sat on the edge of my bed, side by side, as he ran his hands through my hair until I calmed down.

Although my first semester grades haunted me throughout the spring, Taylor continued to build my confidence. He was unlike anyone I'd dated in the past, making our relationship a priority. We frequently went out for meals and he slept at my apartment often because I preferred mine to his.

In April, I told him I loved him and he said he loved me, too. This was a first for me. In many ways, law school wasn't going as planned, but in other ways, it was going very well.

I kept hoping Taylor was right about those initial grades not ending my law school career. Throughout my entire life as a student and an athlete, I'd always started slowly but worked hard and triumphed in the end. Law school would be no different – there was still time.

THREE
SPIRALING

ONCE IN LOVE, my romance with Taylor began having a strange effect on my body. Late one night in April, one kiss led to another and before long, Taylor was taking off my nightshirt.

I lifted my torso to help ease the transition to nakedness and my exposed breasts touched Taylor's chest. A shiver of excitement ran down my spine and a tingling fizzled inside my head, like tiny bubbles popping. Immediately after this sexual sensation, my head and neck flopped backwards against the bed, in a harsh whip-lashing motion.

"You okay?" Taylor asked.

"Yeah, my head just gave out on me, I guess," I stretched my neck from side to side.

The tingling in my head was the same strange signal that usually warned me that I was about to lose my knees. Yet, lying on my bed, my knees hadn't given out on me, or if they had, I hadn't noticed since they weren't holding me up. The wave of weakness was familiar, but something I hadn't felt in my neck. Although I was feeling good – certainly happy – I hadn't been laughing.

As this continued to happen in the bedroom with Taylor, I began calling it my "head thing." When my head thing came on, I warned Taylor and he propped pillows under my head so it wouldn't flop around uncontrollably. Sometimes I suggested that he go on, despite the fact that being sexually aroused left me limp as a ragdoll. I didn't want to stop our sexual encounters so abruptly, but often I couldn't handle the disparity between my desire and my weakness, and asked Taylor to stop. My head thing ruined many romantic evenings that spring.

In addition to laughter and sexual arousal, other emotions began bringing on the melting. One afternoon, I stood on a busy street corner in Boston waiting for the walk signal. When I had the right of way, I stepped off the curb to cross the street and a car inched out toward me, about to turn into my path. I glared at the driver, thinking he wasn't going to yield to me, and with this, my knees buckled. I stumbled slightly before continuing safely across the street. Nothing had been funny, but the slight irritation brought on the same physical feebleness.

A few days later, a young cashier at a grocery store asked if I'd like to donate a dollar to ALS (Lou Gehrig's Disease).

"Yes, please!"

The cashier blinked. "Wow, I usually don't get such enthusiastic responses."

I looked at him. "My uncle died of ALS." My knees melted, then caught themselves. I wasn't sure what I was feeling exactly, yet this communication with the cashier brought on the weakness as well.

The incidents also became more physically drastic. In May, I bent over my friend Edward's computer screen to watch a Saturday Night Live skit and when I laughed, my legs turned to Jell-O. My whole body collapsed and my elbows struck Edward's desktop.

I continued to ask friends and family, even a few people in medical school, if anyone had heard of anything like this. No one had. I looked online, visiting Web MD and searching for information, but couldn't find anything relevant. I promised myself that as soon as exams were over, I'd deal with the problem.

That same spring, while on one of my ritual runs along the Charles River, I experienced a sharp pain in my right knee, like a dagger cutting under my kneecap each time my right leg hit pavement. Later, I went online and learned that this was a common problem experienced by many runners, appropriately called "runner's knee."

"The best treatment is time off," the running websites unanimously advised.

Time off? How *much* time? After a few days of rest, I tried going for a run again but the pain returned. I vowed to give up running for a week. Each day off, my body and mind yearned to flee from school to relax in a sweaty workout. After a week, I double-knotted my sneakers and jogged toward the Charles River, but failed to make it within sight of the water before the acute knee pain resurfaced.

Unable to run, I devoted my time that spring to studying and getting at least eight to 10 hours of sleep a night. I found new tactics to help me stay awake for this round of exams, including making multi-colored flash cards and elaborate hand-written outlines.

I studied in a coffee shop near my apartment, purposefully sitting at the counter next to the barista stand where the drinks were made. The sips of steaming coffee, the scents of fresh espresso grinds, and the constant clatter of cups and spoons were invigorating. Even the conversations of others, something I usually found distracting, were a welcome addition to my studying environment now, since any shifts in energy helped keep me alert.

Late one evening, Taylor met me at the coffee shop, after he'd finished his own studying. He pulled up a chair at my table and quizzed me on

Civil Procedure. He remembered the complex case progressions from his first year perfectly. Talking through the material brought it to life for me and helped move words from the page into my head, or so I thought.

Entering the room for my first exam that semester, my grades from last semester lurked in the back of my mind. I tried to tell myself I was much more prepared this go around. When the exam began, I read the questions and quickly spotted the issues. I knew I had the answers. All I had to do was regurgitate them on the page.

I'd highlighted the answers in my notes, written them in fancy lettering on my flashcards and outlines, yet now I was drawing a blank. Somehow, they hadn't translated into memory. All our exams were technically open book so thankfully my studying materials were close by. As my classmates typed away with familiar gusto, I frantically leafed through my pile of paperwork. The keyboard chorus was in full crescendo, while I sat in silence until I eventually found the answers in my notes. I never quite caught up with those around me.

The day after my exam, I awoke leisurely around 9 a.m. and decided to study at the law school library instead of the coffee shop. I made myself oatmeal and picked up a coffee on the way. I'd perfected my route to school the past year, getting my commute down to 15 minutes, including a few minutes on the highway.

Rounding a large curved entrance road to the highway, a heaviness rolled in over my head like an ominous fog. My eyes burned. The clock in my car indicated that it was a few minutes before 10 a.m., which was strange, as sleepiness almost never touched me this early.

Accelerating to keep up with the other vehicles, the subtle vibration of my car was a sweet soft lullaby. I fought hard to stay alert. Driving 70 miles per hour on a highway was important work. I'd dutifully turned over the past 10 hours to sleep. This was my time – daytime. I slapped myself hard against the face. There was no time for gentleness. *Just… stay… awake.*

Before long, I approached the exit and drove up the ramp toward a large rotary intersection in Newton nicknamed the "Circle of Death," as it is no-toriously known for accidents. Sitting dizzy at a stop light in the circle, the red brake lights of the Jeep in front of me flickered bright to dim, bright to dim. I saw three brake lights, then nine, then six, then three again. Law school was only a few minutes down the road so I continued forward, squinting to make out the road in front of me.

Next thing I knew, I was in the school parking lot with the engine running, the car in park and my seat back reclined. I wasn't sure how I'd gotten there, only that I'd been tired on the highway and followed a Jeep around the rotary. I was unable to recall any visual images of pulling into campus or choosing that particular spot. It was 10:15 a.m. The scenario didn't add up, and for once, my river of reasoning ran dry. With hands gripping the wheel to keep me from shaking, it was clear that my sleepi-ness was not normal.

After exams were over, I began my summer job doing legal research for a professor at school. The commitment was minimal, leav-ing me plenty of free time to enjoy my summer. I hoped that this relaxed schedule would re-energize me – yet instead my sleepiness only got worse.

One morning in early June, I awoke from a perfect night's rest and plunged into doing legal research for my professor at my desk. After about a half hour, tiredness cornered me again. I looked at my bed, still unmade from last night's rest. *No, Julie.* I turned back to my computer to continue working.

Soon, words from the screen spiraled through rollercoaster curves inside my head. Freed from sentences and paragraphs, they swam between con-sciousness and unconsciousness. Sitting upright in my desk chair, two feet from my bed, I drifted off to sleep.

A few days later, I sat alone in my room and logged into the online tran-script program to check my second semester grades. B- in Constitutional Law, B- in Civil Procedure, B in Criminal Law, B in Professional Responsibility and a B+ in Legal Research and Writing. Although not as bad as my first semester grades, my average put me somewhere in the lower half of the class.

For the upper half of the class, GPAs were broken down in a detailed chart so students could indicate on their resumes whether they were in the top 10, 15, or 20 percent, etc. The bottom half of the class wasn't on the chart. I'd thought that putting my GPA on my resume was as important as listing the name of the schools I'd attended, but my career services mentor advised me to omit my GPA since it was better to have an incomplete resume than one so damaging. This was not how I'd pictured things going.

S oon thereafter, I traveled to New Hampshire to visit my father and stepmother, Diana, for the weekend, hoping to get some advice. Dad was my go-to problem solver, always responding with cerebral calmness.

One night in college, after losing my wallet, I called Dad.

"I'm sorry, I'm sorry," I said over and over.

"Julie, it's just *stuff*," he responded. "It's plastic and paper and it's all replaceable. You have your *health* and that's what is most important."

With that, he methodically listed the various steps to take, from canceling my debit card to replacing my driver's license and school ID. I didn't understand why he took the opportunity to be thankful for my health instead of scolding me for being irresponsible, but I was grateful to have a saint for a father. In his mind, there was no challenge that couldn't be overcome.

So, that June weekend, I went to Dad in hopes that he would start picking up the pieces and putting me back together. I left Boston around 8 p.m., preferring night driving, as bright sunlight often strained my eyes and led to sleepiness. Fifteen minutes into the hour drive, a gripping weight came over my skull, clenching my brain. I fought it off and continued driving 75 mph in the left passing lane on I-95 north, repeating: *Just get home, Julie, just get home.*

Nearly 20 minutes later, I started losing touch with my judgment as cars around me faded in and out of my radar. Noticing a sign for Newburyport, I crossed four lanes to take the exit. As soon as I did, I passed a few big gas stations, then pulled into a Dunkin Donuts parking lot and stumbled out of the car. Inside, I ordered a large iced coffee.

Feeling refreshed, I got back on the highway and quickly crossed into New Hampshire. It was a beautiful summer evening, with a silver moon hanging low in the navy blue sky, hovering over picturesque pine trees. It could've been a movie set.

When I tell people I'm originally from New Hampshire, they often respond with bug-eyed enchantment, as if instantly taken back to the first time they laid eyes upon lakes and mountains. Of course, having been born there, these things were commonplace to me. However, now living a hectic city life, I appreciated the robust nature of my "live free or die" roots more than ever.

My eyes began to burn. I reached for my iced coffee and took a few large gulps, but it wasn't helping. I stretched my neck from side to side and slapped my face. When that didn't work, I remembered an old trick from high school.

In 2000, I rode in a friend's Volvo station wagon to an after-prom party on Cape Cod. Our destination was an hour and a half from our high school and it wasn't long before our excitement turned to whispers and yawns. Maybe we'd had enough partying for one night. Maybe we should have turned around and gone back home to bed. Although we all probably thought the same thing, we kept going, riding along in the pitch black, headlights pointing toward Cape Cod.

As I faded to sleep in the backseat, a gust of highway wind struck my face. The driver had rolled down all the windows and now reached for the radio dial, turning the volume all the way up. He started singing along to the familiar '80s tune, "Come On Eileen." His girlfriend, sitting in the front seat beside him, joined in. The other two people in the backseat with me chuckled and we joined in at the chorus.

There was no need to be self-conscious about butchering the lyrics, as we competed for airspace with the much louder roars of wind whipping through the wide-open windows. Earlier that evening, my hair had been curled into careful spirals and cemented with hairspray. This same hair was now twisted into tangled knots. We were all shivering, but no one complained or asked to roll up the windows. Soon, the black air smelled like salt, a sign that our destination was close. We arrived on Cape Cod around 1 a.m., wind-swept and tired, but happy.

Seven years later, driving along the highway in New Hampshire, desperately wanting to get to Dad's house, I rolled down all the windows, found a strong radio signal and cranked up the volume. I tried singing along but didn't know the words to the song. The heaviness remained.

I fussed with the radio dial, looking for a more upbeat song to help fight against my heavy eyelids. I don't remember closing them, only that as they opened, a guardrail was approaching at 45 mph. My car glided up an exit ramp and was about to turn sharply to the left, when I slammed on the breaks. I tried to steer the wheel to catch up with the curve in the road, but my tires swerved. My heart hit the floor, and then, as quickly as I'd lost control, my car's traction returned and continued safely along the ramp.

There were no other cars in sight. I was on the exit ramp toward Dad's house. What if another car had been behind me? I could have put others in serious danger.

Blood pumped through my body with vigor. The moment of terror had pulled my head out of an otherwise impenetrable fog and the rest of the drive was a breeze.

At Dad and Diana's house, Dad opened his arms for a hug. His steady blue eyes calmed me right away. Diana welcomed me with a big smile and hug too. She was good for Dad and I loved her for that. I was happy to see them both. I was safe here. The details of my reckless driving went unspoken. Perhaps the moment scared me too much to internally process it, rendering me unable to acknowledge how out-of-control my life had spun. Whatever the reason, the experience evaporated.

The next night, Dad, Diana and I went to the Olive Garden for dinner. Diana raised her glass. "Here's to Julie for finishing her first year of law school!"

"Hooray," I responded quietly, trying to be polite. I couldn't look up to meet her gaze or Dad's as our glasses clinked. Saying cheers to the biggest academic failure of my life seemed wrong.

"The worst is over," Dad chimed in, perhaps sensing my lackluster response to the topic of law school. I reached for a breadstick.

"And you have a great boyfriend! We're so proud of you." Diana added.

My whole body tensed up. My relationship with Taylor wasn't a consolation for everything else going so poorly the past year. I didn't know whom Diana was talking to, but it certainly couldn't have been the girl sitting next to her at the restaurant. Not wanting to ruin the happy version of me she'd created, I didn't respond. For the rest of dinner, I ate my food, sipped my wine, and said my pleases and thank yous.

When we arrived home, I took off my shoes and started heading to bed.

"Ice cream?" Dad asked.

I stopped in the hallway. "Vanilla?"

Dad smiled. "Vanilla *and* chocolate."

He always stocked the freezer when I visited. Trying to eat healthy, I rarely bought ice cream for myself, but there was something different about indulging at home. I turned around and returned to the kitchen.

"All right, twist my arm."

"Me too, Tom." Diana added from the living room.

Dad pulled the ice cream cartons from the freezer and I reached for three glass ice cream bowls in the cabinet. We piled the bowls with ice cream, topped them off with chocolate syrup and peanuts, and Dad called to Diana to join us at the kitchen counter.

"Dad, remember how you refused to let me swirl my ice cream as a kid?"

"Of course. You wanted to turn your ice cream into soup!"

"So? What was the big deal?"

He shrugged. "I don't know. It just annoyed me."

Usually so patient, it was funny to hear him admit that something *actually* got on his nerves. I glanced at Diana and then Dad, and we all burst out laughing. The tingling in my head came quickly and my neck gave out, dipping toward my chest, lifting up briefly, then dipping forward again. Just a moment later, my head regained strength. Dad and Diana had front row tickets to what must have looked like a convulsion.

"Julie, what was that?" Diana asked.

I winced in reaction to the strange discomfort. "My head thing."

I'd already told them about my knee buckling laughter on several occasions over the past year, but they'd never seen it nor pressed me to see a doctor about it. Now I explained that the weakness had spread to my head and neck.

Diana frowned, "Julie, that's scary. I think you should have it checked out."

I agreed, but where to start? We discussed the incidents in detail. Since emotions seemed to trigger the responses in my body, Diana thought it might be neurological. Next, we talked at length about my extreme fatigue. My sister's husband had sleep apnea, so Dad thought maybe I had something similar – a type of sleep disorder.

I told them about my runner's knee stopping me from running and leaving me feeling sluggish and overweight. Tears streamed down my face when I admitted to being deeply disappointed by my first year in law school. Dad suggested that I meet with the Dean of Students to discuss strategies for improving my grades and happiness at school.

I returned from New Hampshire with a tangible list of issues to address – my sleepiness, the melting in my knees, my runner's knee and my grades. I scheduled an appointment with a general practitioner at health services for July 3, and set up a meeting with the law school Dean of Students for early August. I planned to resolve my problems by summer's end.

FOUR
DISCOVERY

ENTERING HEALTH SERVICES ON July 3, a nurse pointed toward a chair. There was no talk of undressing or wearing a smock. I liked health services already. Soon, Dr. Andrews entered the room. A lock of her silver grey hair caught the light as she smiled and shook my hand.

"Just to warn you," I said, "I have a few problems to discuss."

"Okay, that's fine."

We were eye level and I was thrilled to have the full attention of a wise, older female doctor.

"I'm sleeping all the time recently. I rarely have energy and sometimes I'm even tired in the morning. I think I may have a sleep disorder."

"How long have you felt this way?" she said as she calmly took notes.

I had no idea. Thinking back, I saw myself standing weary-eyed at the bathroom mirror during Property Law class last September.

"A year." My palms started sweating. I hadn't admitted that my sleepiness went that far back until this moment.

Dr. Andrews asked about my nightly routine and I proudly reported getting at least eight to 10 hours of sleep a night.

"Do you snore?"

"I don't think so. My boyfriend has never mentioned any snoring."

She asked me to describe my sleepiness in more detail, so I explained that I was having a hard time getting through classes during the day and my homework at night.

"Most recently, I've been having trouble driving, even short distances in the morning."

"Well, I'm not sure." Dr. Andrews leaned back in her chair. "Lots of people get sleepy while driving. Even I have to stop for coffee sometimes…"

I had no way of measuring my sleepiness against hers to determine if mine was normal or not, I only knew what it felt like inside my head. My gut instinct was that my recent sleepiness was not normal. I wasn't sure, but the smallest voice inside me said, *I don't think this doctor is talking about the same kind of sleepiness.*

"How about you hop on the scale?"

I slipped off my shoes and stood on the rickety old-fashioned metal scale. Dr. Andrews tinkered with the weights until the scale fell even.

"169 and a half pounds."

"169? Are you sure?" I knew I'd gained weight recently, but I'd been wearing loose summer dresses and hadn't realized it had been so much.

"I weighed 155 pounds in April."

The doctor's eyebrows lifted. "You've gained 14 pounds in 3 months?"

"I guess so." I stepped off the scale, still staring at the numbers. This was a first for me. I'd never reached 160 pounds before, and now I weighed almost 170.

The doctor asked about my eating and exercise habits and I explained my workout routine up until the recent change due to my running injury. I was a healthy eater and hadn't changed my eating habits.

Dr. Andrews thought something might be wrong with my thyroid and ordered some tests. She also suggested depression. I didn't feel depressed, I felt tired, but I couldn't fully trust my instincts anymore. We moved on to my next problem – my knees giving out with laughter.

"I've never heard of anything like that before."

"Perhaps it's neurological?" I suggested.

"It could be neurological, and I'll refer you to a neurologist if you really want, but it's probably some strange rare disorder you'll have to get used to."

My throat tightened. It had never occurred to me that there might not be a solution. I'd assumed it was only a matter of getting a diagnosis and then treatment. The image of stumbling across the street flashed in my mind. I couldn't imagine just getting used to it.

Lastly, I told her about my runner's knee and she set up an appointment for me to meet with a sports medicine specialist the following week, on July 10.

I left health services with business cards listing my follow up with Dr. Andrews and my sports specialist appointment. Her plan was to check the thyroid first, then proceed from there.

The next day, the Fourth of July, I attended a rooftop BBQ with Taylor at a law school friend's apartment in the Back Bay. Standing with friends, I sipped white wine from a plastic cup. When someone said something funny, my head tingled and my hand relaxed its grip on the cup, sliding through my fingers. I regained control in time to catch the cup before it fell to the floor.

To my friends, my fumble appeared nothing more than momentary clumsiness, but I knew better. I placed the cup on a ledge, no longer trusting my hands to hold it. Turning my palms upwards, I studied them like a fortune-teller. Something was terribly wrong. Something had shifted.

Later that evening, fireworks lit up the Boston skyline above the Charles River and the Boston Pops played music in synchronization with the light show. Taylor stood beside me, a situation I'd always longed for on past Fourth of July celebrations when single. But now, I was far from him. Bursts of pink, blue, green and gold spread across the dark sky like a gigantic artist's canvas, yet none of it moved me. There wasn't even the slightest spark of joy in my heart. Unanswered questions echoed in my mind and I sensed that my livelihood was wavering in the face of things I could not explain.

A few nights later, on the phone with Taylor, my discontent came up in conversation.

"I'm feeling pretty depressed," I said. The phone line buzzed in silence. "Have you ever felt depressed?"

"What do you mean?"

"Depressed? Have you ever felt so sad that you don't feel like yourself?"

"I don't think so."

"Ever lost your desire to get up in the morning?"

"No."

His succinct responses spoke loudly. Perhaps Taylor had never felt deep sadness or maybe he wasn't introspective about emotions. Thinking about it, I realized that I'd never seen him really upset. He always seemed perfectly content, except for comical moments of minor frustration when the Red Sox lost a close game.

"Shouldn't our relationship be a source of happiness for you?" He sounded exasperated.

"Yes, it should," I paused, "but it's not that simple."

He didn't understand. I wished we could've launched an IV tube between us so he could've passed his happiness along the line to me. In a desperate attempt to help him feel my pain, I thought up hypothetical scenarios of things happening in his life that might upset him but it was no use. I fell asleep lying on top of my bed, mid-sentence in our conversation, with my cellphone sandwiched between the comforter and my cheek.

The next day, I visited health services in the morning to review my test results with Dr. Andrews. She concluded that nothing was wrong with my thyroid and, unsure about what else could be wrong, she referred me for a sleep study.

Dr. Andrews didn't mention my knee buckling laughter and neither did I. After the appointment, I called the local hospital's sleep center and reserved the next available consultation for late July.

Taylor and I had plans to get together that evening but I wasn't feeling up to it. What would we talk about? Our recent phone conversation festered and his inability to empathize with my sadness created a dissonance between us. Perhaps our relationship wasn't as strong as I'd imagined. I needed emotional support and Taylor wasn't giving it to me.

Afraid I wasn't thinking clearly, I called my sister, Michelle. She was seven years older than me, married with two young children, so I often looked to her for relationship advice. She believed it was important for a boyfriend to be able to talk about important things like depression and sadness.

I called my friend Elise for a second opinion. She thought it was only natural we didn't connect about emotions, "He's a guy!" she concluded. "They don't understand that stuff."

I re-dialed Michelle and told her Elise's point. "Trust your gut, Jules." My gut was thoroughly confused.

Taylor called in the afternoon. "What's the plan for tonight?"

"I dunno."

"Should I come over there?"

"I don't think so."

"What's wrong?"

"I think we should break up." It just came out.

"Seriously? Why?"

"I don't know. I'm just so upset with myself right now that I don't feel like I can do it." My justification was flimsy. I didn't know what else to say.

"No, that's fine." He spoke louder than usual. "If you don't want to be with me, that's all I need to know."

"Taylor, I'm sorry."

"I'm bringing you your stuff."

"Right now?" My voice trembled.

"Yes, I want to get this over with."

Our break up conversation was over in less than two minutes and he was on his way with my stuff – the minimal belongings I kept at his apartment for sleepovers. My hands quivered as I placed his sweatpants, t-shirts and bathroom products into a brown paper bag.

In 15 minutes, he was at my door, his face white as a ghost. He wouldn't step inside my apartment, and simply passed me the small pile of my belongings from the hallway. On top was a book I'd given him as a gift. Disheartened, I handed him the shopping bag.

"I'm sorry." I leaned against the doorframe, choked up.

"Well I guess that's it." Anger seeped from every pore. He turned away and didn't look back. I closed the door and burst into tears. This was my choice, yet the emptiness of loss nauseated me just the same.

It was July 7, 2007, and I was lost more than ever.

A few days later, I returned to health services to meet with the sports medicine specialist, excited to get some help with my runner's knee. Part of me thought that maybe the running injury brought on my weight gain and sleepiness, all I needed to do was get back to exercising, and I'd lose those extra 15 pounds and regain my strength and energy.

The young female sports specialist, Dr. Closter, was pleasant, but all business. She conducted a thorough examination of my knee. Her curly blond hair bobbed above her glasses as she twisted my leg various ways while asking a lot of questions.

"Does this hurt? How about now? Any pain walking up stairs? Down stairs?"

In the midst of the intense rapid-fire questioning, she asked, "Do your knees ever give out on you?"

"No," I replied. "Well, yes. There's this thing that happens when I laugh but no one knows what it is. Sorry, never mind, it has nothing to do with my running…" I trailed off.

I expected her to move on to her next question, but she continued to look at me, apparently waiting for me to finish my thought.

I explained the same crazy story I'd told everyone for more than a year in hopes that someone would know something about the melting in my knees.

"I think I've heard of that before," she paused, "It's not my specialty, but let me see." She twirled around to face her computer screen and hit a few keys. I eagerly leaned forward to read over her shoulder. "Loss of muscle tone with emotions, such as laughter, anger…" Goose bumps raised on my arms. Those words seemed to have been written specifically for me.

"Yes, this may be it." She reached for a blank referral form on her desk and began filling it out.

"What is it?"

"Cataplexy. It's neurological, so I'll refer you to a neurologist."

"Yes, please! Thank you so much." I took the paper, staring at the strange word. *Cataplexy.*

We returned to the sports medicine examination and she said she thought I might have tendonitis in my knees. We discussed orthotics and prepared paperwork for X-rays to confirm the diagnosis. Leaving health services that day, in addition to more paperwork, I held the word "cataplexy" in the palm of my hand.

Back in my apartment, I went online and found that, "Cataplexy is the loss of muscle tone brought on by emotions such as exhilaration, anger, fear, surprise, orgasm, awe, embarrassment, and laughter." I gasped and read on. "Cataplexy is a symptom of narcolepsy."

Narcolepsy? I'd heard the word, but I'd thought it was a joke about falling asleep while standing. I'd certainly never nodded off so abruptly like the comical portrayals in movies, but I wondered if narcolepsy accounted for my sleepiness. It *was* a neurological disorder. The dots began connecting. It was like hitting two birds with one stone – explaining both my knee buckling laughter and my extreme tiredness.

In one way, it was as if someone was holding a mirror up to show me the last few years of my life for the first time. My understanding of who I was and how I was living, was changing rapidly. I sat at my computer, clicking through various websites and soaking in the realization that these different parts of my life, things I had not understood, things I had let slip by, were now coming together under the terms "narcolepsy" and "cataplexy."

But in another way, the words on the screen were as meaningless as a magazine horoscope or a fortune cookie. I had no idea what any of this meant; who to talk to about it, or how it might affect my future.

I looked out into the hallway. A powerful stillness filled the air. Jill wouldn't be home for hours. I wanted to scream out the news but knowing that nothing but the inanimate walls of my empty apartment would hear me, I kept quiet and shook in the silence of this lonely self-discovery.

FIVE
NIGHT LIFE

I GRABBED A CUP of tea and settled in to read more. It seemed that narcolepsy accounted for something else that had been happening to me over the last couple of years. Shortly after moving to Boston, I awoke one night to the sound of the front door being forced open. Afraid that someone was breaking in, I tried to sit up, but I was unable to move. I felt like I was strapped to my bed in a straitjacket.

As I struggled, a figure entered my room and rushed directly at me. He wore a dark brown hoodie, hiding his face in shadows. His arms reached toward my head and neck, about to attack me. I struggled to move and get away, but it was no use. My body lay like a sitting duck, a perfect prey. Internally, I shuddered in terror.

A few moments later, my body was released from the invisible restraint. I looked around the room wondering where he'd gone. My heart was racing. I got out of bed and tiptoed to the door, pushing it open slightly to peek into the hallway. There were no signs of any intrusion. Jill's bedroom door was securely shut. I walked to her door and leaned my ear in to listen. All was quiet. How could she not have heard the same disturbance that had wrestled me from my sleep?

I continued to the living room. Our fire escape was attached to the big bay windows at the front of the living room. The windows were securely locked. I replayed the events in my head. I wasn't sure, but I realized that perhaps the break-in hadn't happened. Dismayed, I went back to bed.

After that, I experienced realistic break-ins about once a month. They were all similar, involving ambiguous figures entering and attacking. I was never able to defend myself. Once I could move again, it took me a few minutes to piece things together before concluding that nothing had happened. I told myself they were just nightmares, even though they were unlike any nightmares I'd had before.

One afternoon, I napped on the couch in our living room and awoke to a cat scratching at my arm. His claws moved slowly across my arm, and although it wasn't excruciating pain, it still hurt. I wanted to lift my arm to get away, but I couldn't move, and the cat kept scratching me. When I was finally able to move, I lifted my arm to inspect it for scratch marks. We didn't have a cat and my arm was fine. I quickly realized that this hadn't happened, even though the scratching remained very real in my memory.

Some evenings, I fell asleep on my bed surrounded by law school homework and woke up to Jill coming home. I'd hear her keys jingle in the door and watch her walk into the apartment. She'd proceed past my bedroom to the living room, without greeting me, as if she didn't see me. I wanted to yell out, *Jill! I'm right here,* but I had no voice.

Eventually, I'd regain my ability to move and speak, and realize that Jill wasn't home. I assumed that she'd come home and left, to go to the gym or grocery store. It wasn't a big deal, I was just surprised not to find her there. When Jill returned home later, I'd ask her if she'd come home earlier while I was sleeping and she'd say that she hadn't.

I mentioned my odd visitors to my brother, who was five years older. He said the same thing had happened to him when he was a freshman in college and reassured me that it went away eventually. I figured mine would go away, too.

In June, just a month before discovering the word narcolepsy, I had a particularly strange experience at Dad and Diana's house. I'd fallen asleep on the couch in the den and hours later, awoke to the repeated ringing of the doorbell. From the den, I was the closest to the front door, which I assumed was why no one else heard the ruckus. The ringing was urgent and persistent – a call for help perhaps – an incessant punching at the glowing rectangular box on the other side of the front door.

I thought I'd better take a look at the situation before deciding what to do. However, when I tried to sit up, I found that I couldn't move. I tried to fight the heaviness but it was unforgiving. The doorbell kept ringing, spirals of high-pitched synthesized ding-dongs. *Enough already! I'm coming.* Or at least, *I'm trying.*

After a period of time that felt like forever but may have only been a few seconds, I lifted myself to an upright position. Things got even stranger then. The house was absolutely silent. I looked across the dining room toward the front door. Everything seemed completely normal but different at the same time. What had happened to the doorbell? Why had the person stopped ringing it? Was someone still outside?

I looked down and noticed Sox, Dad and Diana's beautiful white Wheaton Terrier, curled up and conked out by my feet on the couch. It was a picture-perfect moment, something contrived for a cheesy dog-lovers calendar.

She's usually a lively pup, always up for an adventure. So why hadn't she dashed to her lookout post at the front of the house, standing on her hind legs to see out the window? If it were someone she recognized, she'd be wagging her tail by now. If it were a stranger, she'd be barking. Yet she lay like dead weight across my feet. Had she slept through the incessant doorbell-ringing? Impossible.

I realized that when I thought I'd awoken to the doorbell ringing, I actually hadn't. Maybe it was just a dream, but up until what point? I couldn't put the series of noises and actions in an exact chronology.

It was hard to accept that the doorbell was just a dream, because I could still hear it in my memory, like the last song on the radio or an annoying TV commercial stuck in my head. It wasn't a faint memory of an innocuous doorbell – it was an exact "ding dong" sound, with a particular pitch, volume and rhythm. I didn't know which to believe – my clear memory of the past moment or my clear mind in the present moment? Both experiences felt equally real, yet for one to be true, the other had to be false.

Of course, on the night of the doorbell ringing, I was perfectly happy to reach the conclusion that my ears had been lying to me and that no one was outside in the middle of the night. I was comforted by Sox's presence, as she helped me reach this decision quickly before I panicked about the possibility of danger. I fell back asleep with ease, knowing all was well.

I was fast to accept the inconsistencies in my experience, that I was so sure I'd heard the doorbell and simultaneously certain that I hadn't. How could a smart and competent 23-year-old not be able to distinguish the edges of dreams from the tips of reality? How had the picture gone so horribly blurry that I'd looked to a dog to regain my bearings?

At the time, I didn't ask myself these questions. Come morning, I didn't share this experience with Dad, Diana or anyone. There was no need to – nothing had happened.

Now, a month later, sitting across from the word "narcolepsy" for the first time, I saw these night visitors in the light of day. The burglars, attackers, ghosts of my roommate, and doorbell ringer all lined up in my head like a police round-up, a formidable group of thugs who'd been invading my sleep for the past two years. I hated them for creeping in my bedroom and raising a fierce terror in me before evaporating into thin air.

Exploring narcolepsy material online, I quickly learned that, in addition to daytime sleepiness and cataplexy, the two other major symptoms were "sleep paralysis" and "hypnopompic and hypnagogic hallucinations."

Sleep paralysis is the inability to move for a few seconds or up to a few minutes upon falling asleep or waking up. Sleep paralysis is often accompanied by auditory, visual or tactile hallucinations, called "hypnopompic" when at the beginning of the sleep cycle, as one falls asleep, and "hypnagogic" when at the end of the sleep cycle, as one is waking up. I learned that people who did *not* have narcolepsy could have these same experiences too, usually during periods of sleep deprivation or stress, which explained why my brother had them for a period in college. For people with narcolepsy, they happen more consistently.

Many people with narcolepsy described sleep paralysis and hallucination experiences *just* like mine – break-ins, attackers, the inability to move and confusion over what had happened and what hadn't. One woman wrote on a message board that her cat helped her distinguish whether the experience was real or not – she knew that if her cat was still asleep, everything was okay and whatever she felt had happened, was actually a hallucination. I thought of Sox lying by my feet in New Hampshire. The similarities were uncanny. Reading about narcolepsy was bringing situations back to me by the dozen and discomfort I'd repressed and ignored, excused and overlooked.

I had experienced all four major symptoms of narcolepsy – but I read online that not everyone with narcolepsy had all four symptoms to the same degree. Would mine get worse? People identified themselves as having narcolepsy *with* cataplexy or narcolepsy *without* cataplexy. This was all so new and confusing.

I learned that narcolepsy is a neurological sleep disorder involving irregular patterns in Rapid Eye Movement (REM) sleep and significant disruptions of the normal sleep/wake cycle. Sleep had always come so easily to me, it was strange to think that something was wrong with my nightlife. Frankly, I'd never given sleep much thought. It was just a necessary evil that got in the way of my daytime ambitions. In high school and college, I notoriously burned the candle at both ends, which became a huge part of my hard-working persona. Although I never thought I was smarter than others, I was willing to work longer hours than most. For many years, I derived self-worth and satisfaction from actively cheating sleep to get the most out of life.

The more I learned about the sleep cycle and what had gone so terribly wrong with mine, everything began to make sense – from the knee buckling laughter to the night visitors.

The two basic forms of sleep at night are rapid eye movement sleep (REM) and non-rapid eye movement sleep (Non-REM). Normally, sleep begins with Non-REM sleep, including N1, N2, and N3, during which time one's body and mind slow down. In light sleep, N1, one could be awoken easily by noise or outside stimuli. In N2, louder noises would be necessary to wake. In N3, slow wave sleep, it's very difficult to wake someone, breathing is shallow, and heartbeats and brain waves are slow. This decelerating process from N1 to N3 generally takes about 60 to 90 minutes, before REM sleep begins.

All at once, the brain becomes very active and our eyes begin moving quickly from side to side under closed eyelids. The stage is named after these characteristic eye movements that uniquely take place during this period of sleep. During REM sleep, thoughts and emotions flow through the brain, creating the basis of our dreams. Thus REM sleep is often referred to as "dream sleep" since most dream experiences take place during this stage.

During REM/dream sleep, our brain waves look very similar to our brain waves while awake, yet there is a key factor separating dreaming from reality. When our minds enter REM sleep, our bodies become paralyzed (this is called muscular atonia or paralysis of the voluntary muscles). It is believed the body paralyzes itself so that one doesn't act out one's dreams, as this would be very dangerous. Scientists speculate that our cavemen ancestors passed down this paralysis to us – for if cavemen had acted out their dreams while sleeping in the wilderness, predators would've easily been able to find and attack them in the night.

This paralyzed dream sleep state lasts roughly 15 to 20 minutes before the body returns to Non-REM sleep, starting in stage N1 again. The whole sleep cycle revolves like this multiple times over the course of each night, as one's body passes from N1 to N2 to N3 to REM sleep over and over until waking in the morning.

For me, the boundaries between waking, sleeping and dreaming were blurred. With narcolepsy, aspects of REM sleep take place at inappropriate times. For example, when my knees buckled on me as I laughed, my brain confused my feeling of humor with an emotion of REM sleep and attempted to paralyze my muscles for this "dream" – which manifested itself as the dipping in my knees. When sexually aroused, my brain misinterpreted this for REM sleep too, and tried to paralyze my body, resulting in the muscle slacking in my neck.

The sensations of melting, dipping, and giving out were episodes of partial paralysis, pathologically equivalent to the paralysis experienced by everyone, but usually only while unconscious in REM/dream sleep. But I was experiencing this paralysis during the day, while awake and conscious.

Similarly, the inappropriate timing of REM sleep explained the night visitors. While dreaming of an intruder, part of my brain experienced this on a very cognizant level. Usually the brain is not alert while dreaming, yet it seems that the lines are broken down with narcolepsy.

Experiencing these dreams on a more conscious level, I believed I was awake and tried to react. Yet, I was unable to move because I was paralyzed, as I should be in REM sleep, resulting in the feeling that I was wearing a straitjacket. Because of the incredible power of the mind, I vividly remembered these experiences as if they were real. Scientists have discovered that we actually see, hear and feel through our brains. Although the burglars, doorbell ringers, and ghosts of Jill had not been there, I saw, heard, and felt these dreams as if they were real. In a way, I was both wide awake and dreaming.

SIX
RACING

WHEN I RETURNED TO health services for my follow up with Dr. Closter, the sports specialist, I walked with a much lighter step. She greeted me with a quiet smile and slid my X-rays into the light board.

"You'll be able to see it in the picture," she said as she scanned the image. "Yes, here it is."

She pointed to a small area on the X-ray and explained that my kneecap and cartilage were not lined up properly – causing the rubbing, inflammation and ultimately, my knee pain. The process of diagnosing my knee injury as "tendonitis" was satisfying.

Once again, Dr. Closter methodically moved through the motions of the appointment in a calm, constant momentum forward, like a machine, explaining in detail about tendonitis and remedies for it.

While she tried various shoe inserts to find one that would fit my size nine feet, I took her small moment of silence to speak.

"I have to thank you, you were right about that word cataplexy!"

"Oh yes, I meant to ask you about that."

"It turns out that cataplexy is a symptom of narcolepsy, so you actually solved two big problems. Originally, I saw Dr. Andrews because I was tired all the time *and* because of my knee buckling problem."

"That's great." I was surprised by her mild enthusiasm as she continued to sift through foot inserts on a shelf.

"No, really, I can't thank you enough." I wanted to hand her a Nobel Peace Prize or genius grant. I wanted her to feel like a saint or miracle worker, but she simply smiled and returned the conversation to her specialty – my sports injury.

She didn't fully understand what she'd done for me. Or maybe she did, but helping patients was normal for her. After all, she was in the business of healing people. She took it in stride, as if it was normal – even though from my perspective, she'd unraveled the answer to a great mystery that other doctors had missed.

Dr. Closter said I needed to go to physical therapy twice a week for at least six to eight weeks. In all my years of playing sports as a child and in college, this was my first serious athletic injury. I'd never done physical therapy before.

In college, the trainer's office was right outside the squash team's locker room. I used to peek in sheepishly as I passed by on my way to and from practice. Basketball players, wrestlers and gymnasts sprawled across maroon foam tables, reminding me of a depressing hospital ward.

The broken athletes placed large heating pads over their backs and shoulders, wrapped tape around their limbs and secured braces around their knees and ankles. In the back room was a large silver metal witches' caldron, otherwise known as the ice bath. Many of my teammates sat in the ice bath after practice, but the thought of placing even my pinky toe into that caldron of cold made me cringe.

My body had always allowed me to push myself as hard as I liked without consequences. Of course, I never saw this as lucky or special, until now.

Dr. Closter gave me an order for physical therapy at a local center and told me to follow up in a month to tell her how things were going. She was so thorough and involved with my runner's knee, I felt like she actually cared about it, about me.

On the morning of my first physical therapy appointment, I dressed in a sports bra, t-shirt, running shorts, and double-knotted sneakers. Wearing this gear made me feel like an athlete again, even though it was just "dress up." Like Cinderella decked-out for the ball, I got to feel like a better version of myself for a little while.

The office had high ceilings with radiant white morning sunlight pouring in. After examining my knee and reading Dr. Closter's notes, a young, upbeat physical therapist began teaching me a series of exercises, using different weights, steps and a balance board.

The exercises I did in the office were painless and a few were almost fun, but I soon discovered that those sessions were only a small part of physical therapy. At home, I had to do multiple leg stretches, as well as various exercises using heavy ankle weights several times a day.

The day after my first physical therapy appointment, I went to the gym to do my routine. Luckily, the stretching room was in the basement next to the locker rooms so I steered clear of the squash courts and cardio room, my usual hangouts. I laid out my tape, stopwatch, paperwork, ankle weights and a few different medicine balls.

It took me over an hour to do the exercises, while older men drifted in and out doing a few stretches and push ups on their way up to their "real" workout. I envied their freedom to float in and out of the stretch room, before heading upstairs to sweat out whatever they needed. Although I'd originally felt 110 percent committed to physical therapy, it was much more challenging than I ever imagined.

After a few weeks of slight improvement, my physical therapist gave me permission to begin incorporating some light biking and elliptical training into my routine a few times a week. Light was so light that I wasn't even sweating, and the "increase speed" button stared at me mockingly, and yet, during these light workouts, a dull pain still radiated from my knee.

Pampering this injury was disheartening. I wanted to be free to run again, but any hope of a speedy recovery seemed to recede into the distance. On top of it all, I had other medical problems to distract me from my frustrating tendonitis. A close friend from law school had a family friend who was a narcolepsy specialist in Boston and through this connection, I was able to set up an appointment to meet with this specialist, Dr. Larson.

Inside the pristine hospital lobby, people weaved around one another, heading in many different directions. Doctors and nurses glided with ease, sure of themselves and where they were going. Patients moved with caution, hunched over in distress or pain, through uncharted waters. The polished tile floor glistened like ice. Taking smaller steps than usual, I crossed the lobby toward a large bank of elevators, where a sign read, "Sleep Center – 7th Floor."

I flipped through a magazine in the waiting room until Dr. Larson, a thin man in his 40s, standing at the front desk in a long white coat and khakis, called my name. I stood and shook his hand. Soft-spoken and friendly, his calm demeanor put me at ease immediately. He led the way to a small examination room.

Dr. Larson asked me many questions about my sleepiness, the buckling of my knees and my oddly realistic dreams. I spoke quickly, eager to tell him everything. He did not gawk or stare. Nothing I said surprised him. He understood every word, including the ones that surprised me as they fell from my mouth, stringing together sentences I'd never heard myself say before. I even told him about my head and neck giving out on me during sexual moments with Taylor. Dr. Larson responded with affirmations and more questions.

He helped connect more dots for me. I told him about my unprecedented weight gain during the past couple months and he explained that it's common for people to gain excessive weight as the disorder developed, as narcolepsy may slow one's metabolism. Everything that had seemed so freakish and peculiar to the rest of the world was commonplace inside this small examination room.

After much discussion, Dr. Larson said he was confident that I had narcolepsy with cataplexy, but I would need to undergo the official diagnostic test, a 24-hour sleep study to confirm it. He gave me all the information I needed to set up an appointment at a sleep lab.

Lastly, Dr. Larson said that we would discuss medications after the sleep study but asked if I needed any immediate help with my daytime sleepiness. I said I was fine – my sleepiness wasn't putting me in any danger.

Denial is a powerful mind game. I should have told Dr. Larson I needed help with my sleepiness to avoid a potential car accident. Yet, I was still peeling layers of denial away, unaware that I had a long way to go. Although I'd finally pursued my sleepiness with doctors and found the likely cause, I hadn't fully grasped the depths of my problem.

A few days after my appointment with Dr. Larson, I was driving home to my apartment when my head entered a terrible haze of exhaustion. Only a few blocks from my apartment, I pressed on despite the excruciating weight on my skull. I fought to coordinate my arms and legs in accordance with the traffic lights and other cars.

Turning right onto my block, I opened my eyes to see my car drifting toward a car parked on the side of the street. I must have closed my eyes for a second and not fully turned the wheel to make the right turn. Seeing my car's position, I jerked the wheel to the right, over-compensating slightly, but straightening my car nonetheless. Somehow, I managed not to hit anything, but it was a close call.

Back in my apartment, I reflected on the past few days, realizing that I'd been fighting sleepiness while driving virtually everyday. A layer of denial fell to the floor, revealing for the first time that I was spiraling out of control and needed help. I called Dr. Larson's office and he got back to me later that day.

"I know I said I didn't need any help with my sleepiness," I said, "but I'm starting to have major difficulty with my driving."

Once truthful with myself, honesty with Dr. Larson came easily. Given the incidents I described, Dr. Larson was happy to prescribe a daytime stimulant called Modafinil, commercially sold as Provigil, to combat my sleepiness. I was hopeful that it would give me some relief.

As directed by Dr. Larson, I took a half dose of the Provigil for the first two days. I wasn't sure if this amount helped or not, as sleepiness is hard to measure. On the third day, I took a full dose and definitely noticed an improvement in my ability to drive without experiencing extreme exhaustion.

On the fourth day, I noticed a big change. Late in the afternoon, I stood in front of the bathroom mirror, putting on makeup, when I felt a strange sensation inside my chest. It was a Friday and I was getting ready to go on a boat cruise around the Boston Harbor with my favorite band, Virginia Coalition, performing.

Out of nowhere, my heart presented itself as an active participant in my body – a physical thing situated between other organs, surrounded by veins, arteries and bones, pumping blood to the rest of my body. Bah-BOOM, Bah-BOOM.

I wish I could say it was a romantic moment of the heart, falling in love or a first kiss, or even the rush of a rollercoaster. It was no moment of the sort. It was an everyday moment of applying mascara to my eyelashes at the bathroom mirror.

Why I was feeling my heart here for the first time, I didn't know. Obviously, the beat had always been there, but it was much louder now.

I continued with my makeup, applying blush to my cheeks and wondering if it mattered that I felt my heart, thrashing as hard as it was. I much preferred the quiet version to this new, violent presence. *Go away, heart. Simmer down.* But it wouldn't cooperate. Instead, it stayed strong, spasming with fever. Was it beating *too* fast? Never having truly sensed my heart before, I couldn't tell whether this was a normal or racing heartbeat.

I put my makeup brush down, thinking maybe I shouldn't lift my arms above my heart. I stood with my arms at my sides, trying to relax my neck and shoulders. Examining myself in the mirror, I wondered if I was okay. After a brief moment, I decided to try reclining.

Lying down in bed, my heart sat even heavier in my chest and I imagined it crawling up my throat and choking me. I repositioned myself, sitting upright in bed, bolstered with pillows behind my back, but my heart kept going.

I thought of my medication and got up to find the printed information sheet that had come with the prescription bottle. I rummaged through my desk drawer; the sheet was stuffed under miscellaneous papers toward the back. I hadn't read the warnings, contra-indications and side effects before tucking the sheet away. Reading the information for the first time, one of the warnings glared back at me: "If at any time your heart races, please contact medical assistance immediately."

I grabbed my phone and called "Dad's Cell." Dad was not a doctor, he was a lawyer, but he was also my lifeline, a rational problem-solver and my best friend. Surely he'd know what I should do.

"It's up to you, Julie," he said. "If you feel like you should go to the hospital, go to the hospital."

This was not helpful.

Next, I dialed the number for Dr. Larson's office. The answering machine picked up immediately. At 4:30 p.m. on a Friday in the summer, the office was already closed for the weekend. A pre-recorded female voice slowly advised me that, "If this is an emergency, please dial zero to speak with the hospital operator to have the physician on call paged."

I put my pointer finger over the zero key. Was this an emergency? I froze momentarily, but with my heart's next thunderous thump, I pressed down hard on zero. The hospital operator took my information and assured me that a neurologist would call me back shortly.

I paced around my apartment, waiting for the call. In my imagination,

I saw a doctor receiving a message on his pager and immediately dropping everything to race to the nearest phone to dial my number. Reality didn't quite live up to my imagination. I called the hospital operator back, wondering if something had gone wrong. Nothing was wrong. I wondered if I should just go to the hospital.

Finally, my phone rang. It was my sister. She'd talked to Dad and was worried.

"Julie, I think you should go to the hospital."

While on the phone, my doorbell rang. My friend, Emily, who was going to the concert with me, arrived. I told my sister I'd think about it and call her later.

I'd almost forgotten about the concert. Now, in spite of looking forward to this night for weeks, I wasn't sure I should go on the boat cruise. What if something happened while on the water? I envisioned the headline news story in my head: "23 year old dies of heart complications on Boston Harbor. If only she'd been on land, she would have survived."

My phone rang again. This time it was the on call doctor, who sounded my age, not that age should matter, but his young, casual cadence wasn't comforting. I told him my problem.

"It's up to you," he said. "It doesn't sound like you're having a heart attack, but technically, as a doctor, if your heart's racing, I should advise you to go to the hospital."

Was a heart attack the only thing I should be concerned about? I knew nothing about the heart. All I knew was how unnatural my chest felt. I hung up still unsure about what to do.

No one could make this decision for me – not Dad, my sister, friend, not even a doctor. I decided to wait it out and returned to sitting upright in bed. Emily got me a glass of water and sat at the foot of my bed trying to distract me with fun stories about her summer job. I wanted to be distracted. I wanted to be strong and go to the concert.

Around 6 p.m., I realized I wouldn't be able to relax and enjoy the evening unless I knew for sure nothing was seriously wrong. I grabbed my stimulant information sheet and texted Dad to tell him I was going to the emergency room. Emily drove me to the nearest hospital, stopping on the way to deliver the concert tickets to other friends so they could go on without us.

Arriving at the emergency room, I was quickly ushered into a side room for an EKG. Nothing appeared out of the ordinary. That was good news. Next, I was admitted into the back room of emergency beds for more testing. Behind a curtain, I changed into a smock and climbed onto my designated gurney. Within an hour, Dad arrived from New Hampshire, relieving Emily from the waiting room and joining me in the ER. Within a few hours, the noise in my heart quieted down substantially, although the surrounding area of my chest was still tight and inhibited.

Blood was drawn and chest x-rays were taken, but the results of all the testing indicated that nothing was wrong. After seven hours in a hospital gurney on a Friday night, I was discharged without explanation for what had happened. The ER doctors hypothesized that it was related to the stimulant and advised me to cut back to a half dose for the weekend and follow up with my neurologist on Monday.

It was past 1:30 a.m. when Dad drove me back to my apartment. We rode in silence. I was embarrassed that he'd come all the way from New Hampshire for nothing. Although it was late, the Fenway area was still bustling with life – taxis raced by and clusters of revelers frolicked across streets and ducked into bars for last call. Dad pulled up to my apartment and turned to look at me.

"Will you be okay?"

I looked up toward the dark bay windows at the front of our apartment. Jill was away for the weekend and in truth, I didn't want to be there alone. I wanted to ask Dad to sleep on the couch, just to make sure. Instead, I nodded.

"Yeah, I'll be fine."

I hugged Dad goodbye, thanked him for driving down and apologized for the false alarm. Walking upstairs to my apartment, an ugly emptiness filled my body. I thought of Taylor. If we were still together, if I hadn't broken up with him, he would have been at my side now. I wouldn't have had to be alone.

Over the weekend, some friends got word that I'd been in the hospital and called with concern. I explained that nothing was wrong and we moved on to more interesting topics, including stories from their weekend.

First thing Monday morning, I called Dr. Larson. He was surprised to hear about my strong reaction to the standard dosage of the Provigil, especially since this medication wasn't supposed to have the harsh side effects of the other stimulant options available. He recommended that I continue taking a half dose for a week, then try a three-quarters dose, working my way up much slower until I found a dosage that gave me wakefulness without putting me over the edge. Hanging up the phone, I breathed out slowly, releasing a chest full of nervous energy. I was beginning to sense that medication wasn't going to be the quick fix I'd hoped it would be.

That August, I met with the Dean of Students, Dean Wilson, a spunky older woman with stylish grey hair and a button nose. I'd scheduled the meeting in June to discuss my bad grades, which were still making me queasy.

Dean Wilson tried her best to convince me that my grades were not a reflection of my intelligence, but I wasn't listening to that nonsense. I'd succeeded academically in college, why should law school be any different? We discussed my exam preparations and what I might do to improve my exam performance in the future. I'd never met Dean Wilson before, yet she took my concerns seriously and I appreciated her guidance.

After an hour-long discussion, we fell into small talk and I mentioned my probable diagnosis of narcolepsy.

"Narcolepsy?" Her eyes widened.

"Yeah, I met with a specialist and he's almost certain I have narcolepsy with cataplexy. I'm currently waiting to have the 24 hour sleep study for confirmation."

"No wonder you had a hard time getting through your first year!"

"No, no, that has nothing to do with my grades."

"Julie, you don't think *narcolepsy* affected your first year?" There was a hint of exasperation in the Dean's voice.

I clarified, once again, that the two issues were not related. She explained that there had been another student with narcolepsy at the school a few years earlier. She'd worked closely with him. But still, what did she know about me and my narcolepsy?

She offered to help me pick out classes that I would find more engaging and suggested a few professors she thought would be particularly sympathetic to my situation. She even said I could consider taking a semester off if I needed time to adjust. This was completely over the top. I thanked her for her suggestions, but told her none of this would be necessary.

In mid-August, I traveled to New York City for my law school's job fair, to interview with various firms. The night before the fair, I was staying with Natalie, a close friend from high school and college. Natalie was barely five feet tall, with unruly blonde hair, yet her personality was by no means little. She was a ball of energy, jokes and fun.

As we entered the elevator in her apartment building, she asked if I remembered Celine.

"Of course! How could I forget Celine?" I replied.

When Natalie and I shared a dorm room our sophomore year at Brown, we often blasted music late at night from Natalie's high-tech speaker system. Celine Dion was one of our favorites. Shameless about what our neighbors in the dorm might think of our music choice, we stood on our desk chairs and sang along – sweepings our arms with dramatic gusto and using hair brushes as microphones.

Alone in the elevator six years later, we locked eyes and smiled, and I began softly singing, "I drove all night…" – a line from one of Celine's greatest hits.

Natalie jumped in, "To get to see you!"

We were too old for such silliness, but the song brought back fun memories. As I laughed, my head tingled, my knees shot out in front of me, and my back hit the metal wall. I slid down to the floor. Being filled with joy had pressed the "cataplexy" button. While the elevator surged up to the sixth floor, I was on a different elevator ride, going down.

As the elevator door opened, Natalie stared at me. "Are you okay?"

She put one foot in front of the elevator door to hold it open. I couldn't respond right away. I wanted to tell her I was fine, but my jaw gaped open. My eyes fluttered and my head jerked back, hit the metal wall, and then slid forward again. A few seconds passed and I regained my muscle control. I swallowed, breathed deeply and stretched my neck.

"Sorry, sorry…" I slurred, as I scrambled to get up.

"You okay?" Natalie extended her arm to help.

"I'm fine. It's fine. It was just… too funny." My head tingled again at the thought of Celine. I couldn't think of this anymore. We walked down the hall in silence and Natalie unlocked her apartment door.

"Are you sure?"

"Yeah, I'm just really tired."

On my way to bed, I looked at my formal suit hanging in Natalie's room, ready for the next morning. What if the weakness struck me during an interview? At least I would be sitting. My stomach knotted at the thought of cataplexy invading my interviews. *This illness will not hinder my professional life as a young attorney*, I told myself, hoping that if I said it, it would make it true.

   Luckily, by morning, my strength was restored and I didn't feel any cataplexy during my interviews. At least for now, my cataplexy only existed in small pocketed moments, witnessed by me and a few friends and family. Stealing bits of life here and there was fine. I could handle that. Yet, the incident in Natalie's elevator haunted me. It was the first time I found myself on the ground in a somewhat public space, resting my disobedient arms and legs in the dirt and grime of an elevator floor, and calling the spot "safety."

SEVEN
BEHIND DOOR C

A FEW MILES FROM downtown Boston, atop a steep hill on Commonwealth Avenue in Brighton, stood a dark abandoned office building. The address on my directions matched the address on the building, but I could hardly believe that *this* was what I had been looking forward to for the last month. The parking lot was deserted except for a few cars, so I pulled into one of the many free spaces.

I was on time – 8:30 p.m. on Monday, Sept. 2, 2007. With an overnight bag and textbooks in hand, I walked to a dimly lit bank of elevators. The exposed concrete building looked like it was about to crumble; dried out and broken down. One of the elevators was under construction, so I waited for the other one to slowly make its way to the ground floor, all the time contemplating turning around, getting back in my car and driving home. This place seemed unsafe. This place was also expecting me, and I couldn't wait any longer to get what I needed – an official diagnosis of narcolepsy.

The diagnostic test, a 24-hour sleep study, was hard to book. Dr. Larson had recommended a certain sleep lab; one with a month long wait. At this point, I was confident I had narcolepsy with cataplexy. I was here to satisfy formalities. Young and healthy not so long ago, I now waited to take an elevator toward becoming certifiably sick and tired.

There was a small sign inside the elevator indicating that the sleep center was, in fact, inside this strange deserted office building, on the fifth floor. I hugged my textbooks to my body for comfort. Inside the sleep center, an older gentleman in scrubs greeted me with enthusiasm. This was Ed, the sleep technician who would administer my test. I gave him some paperwork and he handed me additional forms to fill out.

"You'll be behind Door C for the night," he said.

Ed's job seemed conflicted. He was partially running a science lab and partially running a bed-and-breakfast. He ushered me into my room for a quick tour. There was a bed, a chair, a linen closet with extra pillows and blankets, a bathroom, and a small wall-mounted television. The room was self-explanatory, and very stark.

Ed left me to finish my paperwork and change into my pajamas. Everything was pleasant and clean, but something was totally off about this place. There were no windows. The red and brown flower-patterned bed spread was reminiscent of a Holiday Inn, but the massive machinery next to the pillows quickly reminded me this was no holiday.

One of the questionnaires asked me to rate different things: "What is the likelihood that you will fall asleep watching a movie?" Very likely. "Reading a book?" Very Likely. "At a social event?" Not likely. And then a question that caught me off guard: "Do you have muscle weakness with emotions?"

This was the first time I had seen these words in print – the great mystery of my life on a piece of standard paperwork. I checked "Yes" and read it over again. This little phrase, "muscle weakness with emotions," sat casually in my lap, among other phrases, as if it had always been there and hadn't eluded me for the past two years.

The questionnaire had probably been printed out, photocopied and read many times over, with others checking "Yes" too. It was only a piece of paperwork, but it made me realize I wasn't alone. Although I read that narcolepsy affects one in every 2,000 people in the United States, about 200,000 Americans and 3 million people worldwide, I'd never met anyone with narcolepsy. It occurred to me then that others could be close by in Boston.

The sounds of intercoms filled the air, as Ed communicated from his station with the other patients in their rooms. I hadn't seen anyone else, but heard their gurgling mumbles through the walls. Here we were, the sleepy preparing for bed.

Ed returned and took me to another room to get "suited up." I reclined in a dentist-like chair as Ed methodically attached electrodes to my scalp. A static-laden radio broadcast the Red Sox game in the background. Between instructions to turn my head this way and that, we talked Sox. Complaining about the Red Sox is the default conversation of New Englanders. In the winter, we complain about the snow and in the summer, we complain about the Sox.

A few probes needed to be attached to my legs, stomach and chest. I helped Ed with these, by running the wires down my shirt and pajama pants. This was quite the process and I was getting tired.

Finally, more than 40 probes were securely fastened to my head and body, with wires connecting to a small black box at my waist that would go around with me for the next 24 hours. I floundered back to my bedroom, trying not to disturb my 40 new appendages, and climbed into bed. Ed attached a microphone against my neck, tubing under my nose and a pulse reader on my finger. After all of this, I really couldn't move very well. Thankfully, it was bedtime.

Ed dimmed the lights and hurried back to his command station outside my room. Over the intercom, he instructed me on a series of eye movements that were projecting onto screens in the nearby control room.

"Look up, look down, left, right, again. Now close your eyes and up, down, left, and right. Very good."

"Everything's all set. You can go to sleep now."

With that, the lights magically faded to darkness, as if the Wizard of Oz controlled my little world from behind his curtain. Despite noticing the night-vision camera's green "on" light over-head, indicating that I was being watched, I had no problem falling asleep. Snug as a bug tangled in a web of wires, I was out cold in 30 seconds.

Once I was asleep, Ed's work began, watching the motions of my nocturnal brain, looking for irregular waves in my ocean of sleep.

N ine hours later, there was a loud knock on Door C. I expected Ed, so I was startled to meet Chris, the equally energetic but slightly younger technician who would be administering the daytime portion of my test. I wasn't particularly fond of Chris for waking me up; I could've slept much longer, but I was glad the night portion was over. Surprisingly, the finger pulse reader was the most uncomfortable part of the whole situation. Chris removed the pulse reader, tubing, microphone and some of the probes, leaving me with 26 attachments for the day.

I changed into my jeans and collared shirt and eagerly rushed out to make breakfast in the office snack station disguised as a meager "common area." I wasn't expecting an omelet and soy latte, which I would have loved, but the instant plain oatmeal and decaf coffee were a letdown. Caffeine was off limits during the sleep study.

A few other patients occupied the small breakfast table, but no one was talking. This was my first glimpse of the others who spent the night behind doors A, B and D: two older men and a woman in a wheelchair. The wires attached to their scalps grossed me out, even though I was in the same predicament. We were a family of Frankenstein monsters.

I forced down the bland oatmeal and bitter coffee, then sat in the plastic chair next to my bed. We were not allowed to sit on our beds between naps, for fear that if we touched the mattress, we'd turn to sleep, a line of reasoning that was probably justified. I turned on my laptop only to find there was no wireless Internet access. Trying to read a law textbook made me sleepy within seconds. The hour dragged on until Chris came in and said it was time for my first nap.

I climbed into bed with enthusiasm. He checked that all the wires were hooked up, and told me I could go to sleep. This was blissful, heavenly sleep! But then, 20 short minutes later, there was another loud knock. Once again, I wasn't happy to see Chris. He entered my room, turned on the lights and began asking me questions.

"How long did it take you to fall asleep?"

I had no idea.

"A few minutes?"

Chris chuckled. "Faster than that! You were out before I made it back to my station. Did you have any dreams?"

"Yes, I was playing soccer with my first year law school section. My writing professor was our coach and she was furiously yelling at us, and…"

"Did you sleep the whole 20 minutes?"

"Yes." And I wanted to sleep more. This short nap was less than restful. It hadn't energized me. It only reminded me of my compulsive need for sleep – just a sneak peek of the ultimate release. I felt so teased. Now, I had to get out of bed immediately and somehow stay awake for another hour and 45 minutes, until nap number two.

I turned on the television to find a very limited selection of channels, all playing soap operas. My disinterest in daytime television quickly edged toward physical affliction. Eventually, I found an Antiques Road Show marathon, which got me through the awake portions of the sleep study until Oprah at 4 p.m. I seldom watched TV at home but today, it was a lifesaver. I honestly don't know how I would have made it through the testing without this mindless entertainment.

To break things up, I made countless trips to the common area. Behind the breakfast table was the only small window to the outside world. Beyond an overgrown field of weeds, a typical row of Brighton houses stood proudly in the distance. They were large and boxy, with minimal space between them and no front lawns – just stunted pathways and front doors to multiple apartments.

Many of my law school friends lived in houses like these, only a few blocks from here. This window revealed another world to me: my public world, my friends, and my life at school. We'd started classes the week before, so I was in my second week of my second year of law school.

I thought of Taylor, who lived a few blocks from here. Last week, we saw each other at a softball scrimmage and started talking again. It became clear that we both still had feelings for each other, and although nothing was official yet, we'd spent a lot of time together during the past week. I hoped we'd start dating again soon. The last few months had been lonely, facing so many changes on my own. Of course, I had friends and family for support, but a boyfriend was different. I missed his unflinching devotion. Although this was the same devotion I'd tossed off like an itchy cardigan earlier in the summer, I now craved his warmth more than ever.

I thought of my own apartment a few miles down the road. The week before, Jill had moved to relocate closer to school to reduce her commute. We vowed to stay close friends, but my eyes still welled up with tears watching her pack.

The following day, a friend from law school, Tracy, moved into Jill's room. Tracy's long blonde hair had intimidated me when we first met, but we bonded over our mutual love of dancing and law school softball. I thought we'd make good roommates, but the change added to the sense of uncertainty ahead.

The window to the outside also reminded me of school. I was supposed to be in a "Civil Motions Practice" class this afternoon, with a Superior Court Judge. It was a popular and practical class, teaching us skills we would use as young associates at law firms. Filled by third year students, I was the only second year student in the class and lucky to be in it at all, but I was missing class today for *this*. I longed to be out there, instead of in here, a slave to sleep. However, in only a few hours, I'd exchange Frankenstein for normalcy.

By the end of my 24 hours, I was totally exhausted. I'd taken five short naps, and struggled through five excruciating 105-minute awake segments. All I had to show for it was some crusty gunk in my hair where the electrodes had been attached. The elevator slowly brought me down to the parking lot, and back to my reality.

Tracy was home when I arrived at our apartment just after 9 p.m. I headed straight for the shower, scrubbing hard at the sticky gel along my scalp, trying to cleanse myself of the entire experience. I needed to put it away for now. It would take three weeks to get the results of the study, and it was time to return to my law school world.

During my 24-hour hiatus, I hadn't done any homework. I had class at 8:30 a.m. the next morning, a job interview at 1 p.m., and I was unprepared for both. I leaned my head back in the shower, letting hot steam envelope me. I had to trust that my enthusiasm for my to-do list would reignite by the time my alarm went off in the morning.

Thankfully, enthusiasm wasn't my only inspiration. The usual list of law school fears were nipping at my heels as well – a fear of being called on in class, a fear of not getting a job for the summer. These were enough to guarantee that I'd be up early, frantically hurling myself back at the life I'd carefully planned years earlier.

EIGHT
UNDERTOW

S OON AFTER MY SLEEP STUDY, Taylor and I officially got back together, quickly making the transition from estranged exes to love birds, as if the past few months had never happened. Perhaps the only obvious change in our relationship was how significantly worse my loss of muscle tone had gotten since he had seen me last in early July.

Over the summer, I'd collapsed multiple times: in the New York City elevator with Natalie, on a busy sidewalk on Nantucket, on the corner next to my apartment, and many times at home.

When Taylor came to my apartment soon after we started dating again, he made a funny comment as I crossed the living room. My legs buckled and I put my arms down to catch myself, falling into a crouching ball position. He quickly rushed forward to hold me.

After falling, I regained my ability to hold myself up again, but stayed crouched in this position for a few seconds, resting in Taylor's arms.

"It's gotten much worse," he said quietly.

I shook my head in agreement and broke into tears. Taylor rubbed my back until I quieted down. We didn't speak of it after this.

In the weeks following my sleep study, I barely thought about my impending diagnosis. Living on the verge of disaster was a good way to lose track of time. I operated in high gear, scrambling to read my homework assignments and prepare for interviews.

It was officially "interview season" of second year, so everyone around me was just as caught up in his or her own tornados. Interview season was total warfare, as the masses of well-qualified, type-A students emerged from the basement of the law library, armed with their first year GPAs tucked neatly into leather portfolios. Everyone lined up, virtually, through an online program called OCI, to play musical chairs for the limited spots at prestigious law firms. There were job fairs, practice interviews, networking opportunities, information sessions, firm-sponsored cocktail parties, luncheons, dinners, initial interviews, and most importantly, "callbacks." We were encouraged to participate in all-of-the-above.

During this time, second year students floated in and out of classes dressed in formal business attire. It was an exciting time for students and teachers alike, as the buzz of who would be interviewing at which firms was as constant and unavoidable as breathing. I got goose bumps seeing my friends and classmates dressed up for the careers we'd come to school to pursue.

Just a few weeks into school, Friday, Sept. 14, 2007 marked two very special occasions: my 24th birthday and the annual law school boat cruise. Walking the rickety tin plank to board the boat, the other passengers' eyes were on me like static cling. I wore a hot pink dress, aviator sunglasses and the most extravagant Happy Birthday tiara – with gobs of glitter and a fan of feathers six inches high, a gift from my gracious friends who knew me all too well. I was never one to shy away from being the center-of-attention, no matter how aggressive the fashion statement.

Although Taylor didn't come on the cruise, my close friends from law school, and a few of my best friends from outside law school, including my best friend, Sophie, all surrounded me. I was excited about Sophie's recent move to Boston and us being together again. In college, we were on the same squash team and quickly became good friends on and off the court. By our junior year, we were inseparable, always laughing and finding the "gooooood times," as Sophie said, in every occasion. I was about to be the birthday princess of the cruise and having her by my side made everything perfect.

Once on board, I made my way to the boat's top deck, in time to watch dusk turn to darkness. I'd been on many cruises around the Boston Harbor – they were all the same, yet I had never grown tired of these few hours of slight detachment from the city I called home.

There were no clouds that night, so under a dense bed of stars, the view of Boston was spectacular. Perhaps it was the unique vantage point that grabbed so tightly at the muscles in my throat. The boxed lights of the Financial District and Seaport were clustered together tightly, and mimicked in the black harbor waves, which acted as a choppy expansive reflection pool.

Sophie pulled me to the bar for a birthday drink of my choice – a vodka cranberry. I hadn't been drinking much recently, since my cataplexy was sometimes worse the day following a night of drinking, but within the context of my festive birthday celebration, muscle weakness felt a million miles away. I stood tall and smiled ear to ear.

"Cheers to another great year!"

The best part of the cruise came midway through the night, as our boat slinked ever so slowly by the banks of Logan Airport in East Boston. With the airport situated directly next to the Seaport, most planes approached the landing strip from over the water. Standing on the upper deck of the boat with Sophie and other friends, I watched a plane drop lower and lower, and when it seemed as if we could have stretched our arms out and touched its smooth belly, the ground rose to catch the plane, welcoming the night travelers to Boston.

I'd flown in and out of Logan countless times in my life, and yet my stomach dropped every time my plane skimmed over the Boston Harbor like that. Three planes passed directly above our heads – the roar of their engines was loud enough to pause conversations and halt flirtations. Each time, I turned my head toward the sky and dipped back ever so slightly, pretending to slip under a limbo bar.

There was something invigorating about this – I couldn't help feeling small and insignificant as the aircraft brushed over the feathered tips of my tiara, completely indifferent to my existence. After each plane's passing and landing, I quickly regained my sense of entitlement out at sea. Beyond the boat's thin red railings, we floated in the ice cold frothing Atlantic, yet from the top deck, I stood on sturdy ground.

I danced and posed for pictures, holding tight to my tiara and camera, above all my other possessions. In the spirit of celebration, I lost track of my drinking as friends continued to treat me to birthday spirits. The images grew increasingly out of focus toward the end of the night as I wandered aimlessly – the princess aboard her birthday chariot. I lived for nights like this.

The next morning, I woke up with tiara glitter pressed into my arms, chest and shoulders, an indication that the previous night was a wild success. Slowly lifting my bedazzled body off my bed and rubbing my throbbing scalp, I knew I was going to pay for last night's fun today. On my way to the bathroom, I remembered Sophie and I dipping under the planes on the boat and chuckled.

Without warning, my feet tripped over each other, as my left shoulder hit the hallway wall, and after a brief, convulsive fight against the inevitable, my knees sunk to the floor, with my left hip and the palms of my hands right behind them. The weakness moved through me in waves. My neck let go and my head swung around like a tetherball.

As I fell, I tried to let out a cry, but my jaw had fallen off its hinges, so all that came out was a mumbled groan, which didn't reach Tracy on the other side of her bedroom door. My eyelids fluttered and closed.

It was as if someone was playing a prank; pulling a rug out from under me. My body was playing a trick on itself.

I certainly wasn't laughing anymore, as I lay like a haphazard stack of bones on the floor, unable to speak or move. Inside this lifeless body, my mind remained steady and clear, aware of my surroundings and taking in my fall all around me. I could feel my strange position, and although I didn't like it, I simply couldn't do anything about it.

My ability to move had been taken away from me, peeled out of my grip by that strange word "cataplexy." It demanded that I give up the reins, and see life from the ground.

I remained on the floor for about 30 seconds, experiencing my existence through my mind's eye alone as each second passed slowly. I was completely unsure of my physical self and where it stacked up in the bigger game of life. This wasn't the first time I'd fallen to the ground. Although I'd come to know the feeling of falling, this was my worst and longest paralysis yet.

Unable to command my own body, I couldn't help wondering what I needed most to "continue on" in the simplest sense of the phrase. Two things came to mind – my breath and my heart. Those two things, thankfully, were still moving, in what otherwise felt like a corpse. But even my breathing was not really my own. My lungs rose and fell, but it was a much simpler process. I tried to breathe deeper, yet my trying made absolutely no difference. I simply received the shallow breath that was given to me.

After what seemed like a lifetime, I regained life in motion. Starting in my fingertips and resurging through my arms and legs, my strength returned as quickly as it had disappeared. Like lifting up the wooden controller of a marionette doll into the air, the strings behind my neck, arms, and legs tightened to upright attention.

The dots reconnected between my thoughts and my actions, restoring a sense of continuity, of line, of backbone. I raised myself up slowly, all too aware that the balance was delicate, and frightened that if I moved too quickly or experienced another emotion, the scale might tip back out of my favor.

Once on my feet, I returned to my morning activities, but it wasn't long before the weakness swelled again, which was unusual. It had never returned so quickly during the same day. Unwilling to take any chances, I strategically landed myself on the couch in the living room.

After a short rest, I gave it a second try, raising myself up off the couch to cross the room. I walked only a few steps before faltering, as if attempting to cross a tight rope high in the air. I quickly returned to the couch.

I looked around the cozy living room I'd known and loved for more than two years, this space was far from home now. It was an obstacle course of various woods, fabrics, metals and glasses – unforgiving corners, tabletops and chairs. All these objects lined the edges of an even more formidable open space in the middle of the room. The same spaciousness that had originally attracted me to this particular apartment now appeared like a bottomless abyss of quicksand. I asked myself, what if it happened out there, in the middle of the room? There would be nothing to break my fall.

I'd promised to drive Tracy to the airport later in the morning, but there was no way I could be sure of myself behind the wheel today. My arms and legs could turn to spaghetti at any second. When she woke up, I explained the situation and asked her to get my phone from my bedroom. I called Taylor and he offered to drive Tracy to the airport and then come stay with me.

Returning from Logan, Taylor picked up take-out from a local restaurant. We were scheduled to attend a BBQ at noon and a birthday party in the evening, both of which were out of the question now. These were events put on by good friends, people who consistently attended my events; friends who would notice my absence. It pained me to cancel, but there was no way around it.

Of course, on some level, this was my fault. Having so much to drink the night before had clearly made my cataplexy much worse. I hadn't realized it could get as bad as it was. My mind raced through the many possibilities. What if today had been a school day? What if I had an interview scheduled? Luckily, it was only social occasions I had to cancel.

I slept on and off all day while Taylor entertained himself watching movies and sports. Eventually, I texted my friends to flake out on my commitments to their parties, offering vague excuses of not feeling well. They were disappointed but understood. Part of me wished they knew the truth, and that they could see me like this and *really* understand.

Taylor reminded me that people back out of plans all the time.

"It's not the end of the world, Julie."

He was right, but it just wasn't me. I considered myself a reliable friend. When I said I would be somewhere, I was there. Today was an exception.

When it was finally time to go to sleep, Taylor slid one hand under my knees and the other across my lower back, lifting me up off the couch to take me to bed. At six feet, he held me high above the floor and furniture. I knew he was strong, but now I realized how strong. I was dead weight, a pile of bones with spasms of muscle strength, but he carried me with grace and ease.

His legs stretched out, one in front of the other, crossing the living room and hallway into my bedroom, the same space that was impassable for me. His arm muscles tightly contracted underneath my thighs and lower back. My feet swayed in the breeze and my arms rested on my stomach. His body was so consistent, never weakening or giving out for even a split second as he carried me to safety.

Once over my bed, Taylor gently set me down. The bed held me now, I was okay here. I offered a slurred apology and thank you. Taylor turned to go to the bathroom and brush his teeth. As usual, he'd risen to the occasion out of a mysteriously deep place of love and kindness.

He'd seen more of my cataplexy than anyone else, but he rarely addressed my health. He looked through it, either not seeing it at all, or choosing not to inspect it too closely.

Sometimes I probed him for an opinion or reaction. He responded with shrugs and nods, not exactly what I was looking for. What was I looking for anyway? Perhaps reassurance that someone else was bearing witness to this insanity. Or maybe I was desperate to hear that he still loved me, even at a time like this, when I could barely touch upon the nerve that loved myself.

I don't know what I would have done without Taylor that day. I was grateful for his help, yet the dependence scared me deeply, and I imagine it scared him too. Maybe I wanted to hear that I wasn't the only one who was scared. I didn't want to be a freakish stranger in my own body. I wanted to be the same Julie as before, and hoped that having the same boyfriend would keep me attached to my old self.

Regardless, I took solace in knowing that this was all temporary. I would be meeting with Dr. Larson in three days to get the results back from my sleep study. It was the key to medication, recovery and my return to life as I knew it. Hopefully, I would never sacrifice another day to this strange sickness. Hopefully, no one would ever have to carry me again. I held tight to these hopes with a white knuckled grip. I saw no other possible way out. I'd never met anyone with narcolepsy, or any serious chronic illness for that matter. In fact, the words "serious chronic illness" weren't in my vocabulary yet.

At the time, I knew sickness as either small or big. Small sicknesses came and went without making any major impact on life. Up until now, these were the only kinds of illnesses I'd experienced personally – broken bones, tooth cavities, sinus infections, and so on. Things that healed, got fixed, and went away.

And then, of course, there were big sicknesses, like cancer and AIDS – monsters still tightly holding the wool over doctors' and patients' eyes. Big sicknesses did more than impact life, they ended life, the ultimate tragedy. Narcolepsy was certainly no monster, no tragic ending, so it had to be something small, I told myself, something that could be fixed, something that would go away.

When Taylor returned from the bathroom, I decided to hold off on the self-deprecating round of compliment-fishing. We were both ready to put a second bookend on this day. I was asleep before his head touched the pillow, easily swayed by the undertow, back into the fitful sea of dreams and nightmares that would deliver me, washed up, to the next day.

NINE
PRESCRIPTION
FOR CHANGE

MONDAY, SEPT. 17, I was in my gray J. Crew suit before dawn. The next day, I would get the results back from my sleep study, but Monday was the Philadelphia job fair. Although Boston felt like home, Philadelphia was a city I could see myself in, so I'd signed up for our school's job fair there.

It was an hour drive to Providence to catch my 6:30 a.m. flight to Philadelphia. I had three interviews scheduled, so I spent most of the day in transit and in Starbucks. By the time I reached the reception area of the third and final law firm, my suit was wrinkled and my enthusiasm was low. I was ready to go home. The firm's deep maroon walls were the color of a good glass of red wine. Luckily, the modern black leather couches were stiff and uncomfortable, keeping me alert while waiting for my interviewer to fetch me.

A tall thin red-haired woman in her early 50s greeted and escorted me into a sleek conference room. About 30 tall black leather swivel chairs lined the edges of the long mahogany conference table. My interviewer chose two seats for us at the corner of the table.

From my seat, the view of the city caught me off guard. Rows of sunlight lay like sheets along building walls, across street corners and over treetops. I wasn't sure I belonged here, high up in this impressive Philadelphia skyscraper, looking down on life from above.

"Why Philly?" she asked.

This was the most popular question of the day. I could have made up a story about having family in the area or a boyfriend in business school here, but I wasn't good at blatantly lying.

"I really like Philly and consider it similar to Boston, with great restaurants and museums."

I could tell that my motivations weren't moving my interviewer, as she pursed her bright red lipsticked lips, the only color painting her otherwise pale face. Oddly enough, I sensed that, within this context, it would've been less awkward to lie and get the answer right than tell the truth and get the answer wrong. Supposedly, Philadelphia has an inferiority complex to New York City, and law firms in Philly fear that young professionals interview there only as a backup to the Big Apple.

Soon, it was my turn to ask questions. I'd researched their website, read news clips and department descriptions, searched for questions to show that I'd done my homework. Question asking was very important; as it was one of the things I would be judged by, one of the tools used to weed the law student garden.

I began reciting my memorized inquiries about pro bono work and the firm's commitment to diversity. I tried to take the interviewing game seriously, but I was growing increasingly tired of the games: the pawns, the squares I passed through, the squares I landed on, the race to the finish, the inevitable loss to a luckier player.

After running through a few of my planned questions, I decided to break my script and ask one out of personal curiosity.

"You seem like an inspiring example that women really can do it all. What's it like being a high-powered female in a firm like this?"

Any spark between the two of us died instantly. She looked me over for a prolonged second. I should have stuck with my script. On paper, this attorney was everything I wanted to be when I "grew up." Although statistics showed women were leaving law firms at much earlier ages than men, she proved that anything was possible and I looked up to her for it.

When she began to respond, it became apparent that she'd decided to break from her script, too. She explained that she *couldn't* do it all, that she was a mother of three and wasn't always there for them. She wasn't sure it was the way to raise children, however, "You make your choices and live with them," she said. It was an uneasy ending to the interview, but my half hour was up.

I held out as long as possible before passing over my transcript, knowing it was the torch that would incinerate my chances of working here among the wine-colored walls high above Philadelphia. I didn't expect to ever hear back from this woman, and I never did. Back in Boston by midnight, I was asleep before I had a chance to think about what lay ahead the next day.

On Tuesday, Sept. 18, at 12:45 p.m., I stood at the front of East Wing 115, about to give a portion of a presentation for the Intellectual Property Group that I was leader of this year. This was the same underground coliseum where my first year Property Class had been held. Before this day, I'd never stood in the spotlight of one of these large classrooms. I'd always been in the audience.

Looking into roughly 50 blank stares peering at me, my knees shook uncontrollably as I began my portion of the speech. I wondered if the audience was listening to my words or watching my childish nerves getting the best of me. In an attempt to look presentable and professional, I'd worn high heels and a business skirt. If I'd worn pants, no one would have seen my nerves. I charged through my speech, forgetting a few important points and never asking if anyone had any questions. I handed out information sheets and darted out of the room by 1 p.m., leaving my co-leaders to finish where I left off. I had somewhere else to be, someone else to be.

It was a 15 minute drive between being a leader of a law student organization and a neurological patient. I made the trip with ease, reaching the hospital in plenty of time for my 1:30 p.m. appointment. Still wearing high heels and a skirt, I moved slowly across the shimmering tile floor of the hospital lobby, heel-toe, heel-toe, to the bank of elevators and finally to a small examination room on the seventh floor.

"Are you usually this anxious?" Dr. Larson asked.

We'd only been together a few minutes. I was still getting my bearings on this new examination room. I didn't think he was even paying attention yet.

I repeated his question to myself. It seemed he already had his answer, that I was anxious, and had delivered it in the form of a generalizing question. I wasn't sure how to respond, especially since I didn't feel anxious. Then, I remembered my knees. Silly me. On the seventh floor of the hospital, law school had fallen away, if only for a moment.

"Oh, I gave a big presentation at school a few minutes ago. That's probably why – why I seem anxious."

I looked down at my knees. They weren't shaking anymore. I wondered what he was seeing that I didn't.

"Do I really seem *that* anxious?" I asked.

"Just curious," Dr. Larson said. "You seem slightly on edge. I want to be sure the daytime stimulant isn't too strong."

I wasn't sure if it was the stimulant or me. Frankly, I wasn't sure what "me" was anymore. It was as if I'd climbed out of a cave for the first time in years and someone asked me if it was usually this bright outside. I had no idea.

Dr. Larson calmly reached for my folder of records and the dissonance between us crystallized. For him, this was all routine. For me, this defined anxiety. The hospital, the little room, the plastic model brain sitting on the windowsill, his impressive credentials, the folder, the results. It was not every day I sat in a room with a doctor holding my health in his fingertips. Actually, I was surprised my knees *weren't* knocking.

Dr. Larson pulled a single piece of paper out of my folder – displaying a few graphs and charts. His eyes lit up. He was excited by the results of my sleep study, though not in a good way, not that I'd expected good results. No, I needed these bad results, since they were the only way to get closure, the only path toward the beginning of the end of this illness. I just hadn't expected my results to be *so* exciting to Dr. Larson, in the unhealthiest way possible.

He explained that my sleep study results indicated "textbook" narcolepsy with cataplexy. It was the daytime naps where my brain was so impressive.

"You reached R.E.M. sleep in all five naps!" Dr. Larson's eyes popped larger and larger with each word, indicating that, for him, this was all very interesting.

Normally, it takes people about 60 to 90 minutes to reach REM sleep, so they wouldn't enter this stage during a 20 minute nap. People with narcolepsy often enter REM sleep soon after falling asleep. If a person enters REM sleep in two or more of the five naps in eight minutes or less during the study, it's highly suggestive of narcolepsy.

Having reached REM sleep so rapidly and spent so much time in REM sleep during all five of my naps, my results astounded Dr. Larson. He was hoping to share my statistics with other specialists to show younger neurologists what textbook narcolepsy looked like on paper.

I studied the page's lines, numbers and letters that didn't form words. Unfamiliar with the many acronyms used, it was difficult to make sense of this page, never mind trying to draw meaning, excitement or closure from it.

Yet, looking at the same piece of paper, Dr. Larson marveled at the dysfunction inside my brain. Supposedly, it explained everything: my collapsing, my nightmares, and my losing battle to sleep. Here it was – the greatest loss of my life, neatly plotted along an x and y axis. I thought to ask Dr. Larson for a copy of the paper, but even if I took it home, I knew it wouldn't speak to me the way it spoke to him.

Dr. Larson caught himself for a second, realizing this was somewhat of an awkward moment for me.

"Sorry, this may not be as exciting for you."

He said this reminded him of a cartoon he once saw of a man lying ill in a hospital bed and a woman announcing, "Honey, good news! You're going to be in a textbook!" Of course I would rather have been 100 percent healthy than featured on an episode of "Grey's Anatomy," but there was a strange sense of pride in being a scientific novelty.

These results, however good or bad, affirmed that what had been happening to me over the last couple of years was truly biological and neurological, and not something within my personal control, as I had thought for so long. Narcolepsy hadn't changed the way I looked on the outside, besides gaining some weight, I appeared exactly the same. Yet, internally, it had touched my life in invasive ways. Only this paper, striking to neurologists, but unintelligible to most people, myself included, spoke of the greater changes within.

Next on the agenda was medication. Dr. Larson grabbed a scrap of paper and scribbled a few charts, with arrows pointing up and down, and a handful of words and abbreviations. It looked like a basketball coach's game plan. He explained everything slowly and thoroughly – describing the available drugs and how each affected the symptoms of narcolepsy differently.

I listened patiently but as Dr. Larson reached the end of each drug's description, he reported a major complication or side effect. I assumed he was slowly leading up to the good option, the miracle drug, the fix-all. When he put his pencil down and looked at me, I didn't say a word. Was he finished?

It seemed the best medication to get my cataplexy under control was a treatment called sodium oxybate, commercially sold as Xyrem, that I would need to take twice every night – one dose at bedtime and a second in the middle of the night. It would hopefully drastically improve my cataplexy and daytime sleepiness, too. Once starting Xyrem, I'd notice improvements over the next couple of weeks. This sounded hopeful.

"Do you have a roommate?" he asked.

"Yes." I wondered why that mattered.

He said that if a fire alarm were to go off while on Xyrem at night, I might not hear it. Also, this medication was a version of a substance called "GHB." GHB had a long, complex history as a drug of abuse, notoriously known as a "date rape drug" in the 1990s. This information was overwhelming, and yet Dr. Larson considered Xyrem front line treatment.

He described another line of treatment, which was taking antidepressants daily. That also worked well for cataplexy in the short run, however the drugs' benefits tended to wear off over time. Since narcolepsy is chronic, lasting a lifetime, there was a strong chance that my body would grow immune to the different antidepressant treatments over time. In addition, if I stopped taking the antidepressant for any reason, my cataplexy could rebound worse than before. We left this option as a back-up plan and went back to talking about Xyrem.

Xyrem came with lots of rules: no eating two hours before taking the medication at bedtime and no drinking alcohol. Dr. Larson explained that drinking alcohol was counter-productive to my health in general at this point.

I didn't live to drink, but this was a life-changing rule. I'd started drinking in college, so by the age of 24, my idea of a good time was completely infused with alcohol. Partying was synonymous with drinking. I believed alcohol was the spark of fun under my birthday boat cruise, causing me to enjoy the silliness of leaning back to limbo under the planes, giving me the confidence to have conversations with strangers. All this had been strung together by the freedom of drinking, and I honestly couldn't imagine giving it up.

Unfortunately, it wasn't just a question of drinking or not drinking; there was another larger, scarier factor at play – my ability to stand and walk without collapsing. Since I needed to walk more than I needed to drink, Xyrem was the only right choice. The elasticity of life began revealing itself to me on this day. When faced with disabling muscular paralysis, my desire to continue drinking, although closely attached to my sense of livelihood and spirit, didn't matter. It couldn't matter.

Dr. Larson said he was still slightly concerned about the Provigil I was taking to improve my wakefulness. Once out of the emergency room, I hadn't had any other major problems. On occasion, I felt my heart racing in my chest, usually when I got slightly worked up about something. One day during a heated class discussion, my heart pumped furiously. I grew to recognize the sensation and although it was distracting and slightly uncomfortable, I tried to stay calm until it passed.

Dr. Larson explained that the other two stimulants I could choose were notorious for raising heart rates and producing anxiety. I shook my head no to these choices right away. Given my strong reaction to the medication I was already taking, I feared having an even worse reaction to the others. Dr. Larson explained that everyone metabolizes drugs differently, so it might be worth trying the others as a point of reference. I was open to the idea, but not yet. I couldn't afford to risk spending more time in the ER during my second year interview season.

I kept Dr. Larson's scrap piece of paper detailing the different medication options. Even though the graphs were practically illegible, it came in handy during the next few months as I tried to explain my new reality to others. There was something hidden beneath Dr. Larson's soft pencil script – the lack of a cure.

"Are you still interested in art?"

Dr. Larson's question startled me. His unflinching transition reminded me that our discussion was confined to an allotted block of time, otherwise known as an appointment. It was already 2:25 p.m. I found myself trying to drop an anchor on time with Dr. Larson. Given his numerous responsibilities as a prestigious doctor and researcher, this was incredibly selfish of me, yet, for once, I was compelled to linger between these sterile-smelling walls of medicine.

As a child, I answered my pediatrician's questions with the sole strategy of getting a sticker and leaving as quickly as possible. Today, there was no clear exit plan. This hour-long meeting came with a prescription for a lot of change in my life, and I wasn't sure I was ready for any of it. Yet, despite the weight of the words exchanged, time floated on.

"Yes, I am still interested in art." I was curious about where he was going with this. He'd remembered that I was an art history major in college and, although I was impressed with his memory, the question seemed random.

"I'm wondering if you would ever consider doing something with art again. I have a friend who works at a museum. I might be able to put you in touch with her."

I thought he might have forgotten that I was in law school.

"I've always been interested in museum work," I said, "but I'm not sure how this would fit in right now, at least while I'm still in *law* school."

"Of course you can be a lawyer. It's definitely possible, but it may be a challenging career with narcolepsy."

I looked at Dr. Larson blankly. A few minutes earlier, this same man had translated my own brain waves back to me, he'd been my interpreter of dreams. Now, he was a perfect stranger. Although a leading expert on the microscopic region of my brain where narcolepsy lived, Dr. Larson certainly wasn't an expert on the rest of me. "A challenging career" didn't scare me in the least.

Dr. Larson told me a story about another patient who was a lawyer. When his narcolepsy and cataplexy developed, he started slurring his words and stumbling around the courtroom. The judges, opposing parties, even his own clients thought he was drunk. He wasn't, of course. This was cataplexy. Now, he's on medication and doing much better. This past year, he argued a case before the U.S. Supreme Court.

"An incredible personal triumph, but it hasn't been easy for him," Dr. Larson said.

I'd never thought of the possibility of having cataplexy in the courtroom, but I wasn't looking to be affected now. If I'd wanted easy, I never would have gone to law school in the first place. Narcolepsy or not, I was tougher than most. He'd see.

TEN
ACROSS MY LIPS

O N THE WAY HOME from the hospital, I called Dad to tell him my diagnosis.

"What do you mean you're going to take a date rape drug? Why do you remind him of a cartoon of a sick man in a hospital?"

"I don't know, Dad." This was all new to me. I thought Dad would make me feel better, but his uncertainties, on top of my own, made me feel worse. We were both lost. I told him I needed to go.

Narcolepsy was getting increasingly more confusing, taking up more space in my life than I'd originally intended to give it. Back in June, I'd made the appointment at Health Services thinking I would take care of my problems over the summer, before the second year interview season. Here it was mid-September and I was in deeper than I ever imagined. The diagnosis was helpful, a major step in the right direction, but the list of questions and concerns continued to grow higher over my head.

Later, I called Mom to tell her the news and that evening, I told Taylor. My friend, Elise and I had dinner plans later that week so I shared the news with her then. I didn't inform many others of the diagnosis right away. It was just one step of many and telling people didn't really change anything.

I'd already begun to realize that the word "narcolepsy" meant very little to the outside world. Even when I chose to tell others, and explained my behavior, I found that for the most part, people were not affected by this word. Toward the end of August, I informed the professor whom I'd been working for all summer about my likely diagnosis and without blinking, he said, "I'm sorry to hear that," and quickly moved on to talk about other things – his son's soccer tournament, the Red Sox, the weather. It was as if I'd told him I had a cold.

Narcolepsy wasn't a "big illness," by anyone's standards, even my own. Yet, I was starting to sense that it wasn't a small illness either. I honestly wasn't sure what to make of it.

The new nighttime drug, Xyrem, was the weightiest part of my meeting with Dr. Larson, but even this did not affect me immediately. This medication had the most highly regulated distribution system in the country because of the drug's history as an abused substance. A very secure process was in place to ensure that the medication wouldn't get into the wrong hands on its way to reaching me. I didn't want to take any drugs, especially not this one, but *wanting* versus *needing* was different now.

Dr. Larson processed my prescription directly with the specialty pharmacy. They, in turn, contacted me by phone to set up two shipments. The first would be a DVD about how to take Xyrem, the second would be the actual medication. Until it arrived, I continued taking the daytime stimulants and switched gears to return to my law school life as quickly as possible.

Two days after my diagnosis, on Sept. 20, after interviewing with 11 firms in Boston, New York and Philadelphia, I put on my favorite black suit with a lavender shell, straightened my hair with extra care, and went to my only callback interview – my only second chance for an offer at the firm I'd worked at between college and law school. It wasn't until after the recruitment coordinator, a women I knew well, scheduled the appointment that she requested my transcript and writing sample.

As I stood in the reception area on the 14th floor of the glass and granite skyscraper in Boston, I was mesmerized by a massive modern painting hanging above a grand marble stairwell. Had it always been there? The background was a dark, stormy, grey with thick streaks of red and purple cutting through at severe angles. It was an unsettling piece, reminding me of the blood and adrenaline thrashing through my chest.

I hadn't particularly liked the time I'd spent at this firm, at least not my actual work of filing papers for lawyers, but now, one year later, I was hoping for a job as a summer associate. I'd imagined it many times, working through the summer and being asked back as a First Year Associate upon graduation. A dream come true.

As I was reminiscing, the recruitment coordinator came around the corner. "Hello, Julie."

We hugged, then climbed the white marble staircase and walked through a familiar hallway. I saw a few old friends, though there was no time to stop and talk. Just time for polite smiles.

After being dropped off at a corner office, I shook hands with the two attorneys, a male and a female, and sat across from them at a large wooden desk. I'd never actually sat in one of these offices before, only rushed in and out to exchange files.

I looked into the eyes of the firm's two hiring partners. As a file clerk, I'd heard their names and shared an elevator with them on occasion, but I'd never formally met either before today. The male attorney looked down at paperwork and spoke first.

"Welcome back, I guess." He sounded puzzled.

"Thank you, yes, it's great to be back!"

With that, there was no further mention of my previous job at the firm. They were ready to begin their questioning.

Having had a plethora of interviews under my belt, I was ready for anything, or almost anything. After about 10 minutes of familiar questions, one caught me off guard. The dead-faced male partner leaned forward.

"So, what happened?"

Intuitively, I knew what he meant. I'd strategized with my career services advisor and rehearsed the answer, but I hesitated.

"You did so well at Brown. What happened in law school?" he followed up.

"I didn't know how to take law school exams," I explained. "The format was very different from my art history exams in college. But I am meeting with my professors and practicing my exam-taking skills."

This was all true, though in my mind, it wasn't *the* truth. I wanted to say, "Funny you should ask because the most extraordinary thing happened to me! My knees buckle with laughter, I have surreal dreams, and tiredness creeps in during the day. I was diagnosed with narcolepsy with cataplexy two days ago."

Of course, I knew that to be considered for this job, this part of me had to lie down somewhere around my feet and stay put. If any part of this story swelled up and crossed my lips, it would have all been over. Narcolepsy was like a typo on my resume, a glaring mistake and an easy reason to cross my name off the long list of eager legal eagles battling to find their futures at this firm.

Much to my surprise, my cover up seemed to go over fine with the two hiring partners. Of course, they didn't have to accept me, but there were no more steps in the procedure from my end. The recruitment coordinator hugged me good-bye at the elevator, explaining that they had one more week of interviews and then the attorneys would meet to make their decisions.

"Expect an answer in about two weeks."

A few days later, the DVD about Xyrem arrived in the mail. That night, Taylor and I watched it together in my living room.

An older woman with white hair dressed in long flannel pajamas was the star of the "movie." We followed her around her house, stood next to her as she prepared her medication in the bathroom, took the two orange medicine bottles to bed with her, and placed them on her nightstand. She climbed into bed, picked up one of the pill bottles and drank the liquid from it. She returned the empty bottle to her nightstand, turned out the light next to her bed, and fell asleep. The screen was dark for a moment, and then, we re-met the woman in the middle of the night as she woke up to take her second dose of medication.

The DVD reviewed the rules about taking the medication. I wasn't allowed to eat for the two hours before the first dose. I wasn't to get out of bed after taking the medication. After two and a half to four hours, I could take the second dose. If I missed a dose, I could not double up on doses. If I didn't have four hours to stay in bed, I wasn't to take the dose of medication. No driving for six hours after taking the second dose. Lastly, the legal status of the drug was discussed – clarifying that sharing the drug with anyone would put me in big trouble.

The next day, the package with medication arrived, and when it was almost time to go to bed, I unpacked the contents – two large medicine bottles filled with liquid, a syringe-like measuring tool, and two empty orange pill bottles to mix the two doses with water. I called Taylor into the bathroom. He was acting as my lab partner for the night. The Xyrem box was covered in warnings and labels. Standing in the bathroom with my make shift drug-mixing station laid out on the countertop, I was thoroughly nervous.

I had tried smoking pot during my freshmen year in college, while dating a guy who smoked it, but stopped soon after we broke up. Marijuana left me feeling out of control and paranoid. I'd never tried any other drugs, mostly because I was extremely afraid of something going wrong.

Now, at the age of 24, the thought of taking heavy drugs repulsed me. Closing my eyes for a split second, I remembered lying on the ground the morning after my birthday, awake in my head but dead in my body. It was enough to overcome my moment of hesitation.

Carefully following the instructions, I placed the tip of the syringe into the opening at the top of the brown medicine bottle and pulled up on the syringe's handle until 2.25 grams of liquid filled the syringe's tube. After I removed the syringe and placed it over an empty orange pill bottle, I pressed down to squeeze the liquid out. I repeated the process again, squeezing 2.25 grams of liquid into the second orange cup.

I measured one-fourth cup of tap water, and poured it into one orange bottle and repeated for the second bottle. Once the medication and water were mixed, I secured the child safety caps on each dosing cup. Holding one of the cups up into the light, Taylor and I watched the two clear liquids, water and medication, swirling around one another.

I took the bottles to my bedroom and placed them on the filing cabinet beside my bed. I looked at Taylor and then the bottles. All the warnings of this being a date rape drug left me uneasy about going under the drug's spell. Taylor's presence was comforting, if anything went wrong, he would be right there.

It was 11:30 p.m., so I set the alarm on my phone for 3:30 a.m., and Taylor set his phone alarm for the same time, just in case. This would be the time to take my second dose. Taylor turned off the lights and climbed over me, to the far side of the bed, so that I was closest to the orange bottles. I lifted one and unscrewed the childproof top, putting the rim of the pill bottle up to my lips to take my first sip.

I'll never forget this moment. As I tilted my head back and let the liquid cross my lips, slowly slithering along my tongue and down my throat, I gagged slightly. It was the most repulsive substance I'd ever tasted – potent and harsh. Dr. Larson had warned of a slightly salty taste, but there was nothing "slightly" about this. And "salty?" What flattery. Chips are salty – this was nasty. I'd taken a fair number of strong alcoholic shots in my day

– shots that burned the back of my throat and sent shivers down my spine. The contents of this innocent-looking orange pill bottle combined all that and more. I winced and shuddered uncontrollably.

"What's wrong?" Taylor asked.

"It's absolutely disgusting! UGH."

Closing my eyes, I drank the rest of the liquid in the pill bottle and sunk down into my pillow to sleep.

Before long, Taylor was shaking me. He was standing next to me, holding the second bottle. Both alarms had gone off, but I hadn't heard them. It seemed like I had just taken the first dose. It was hard to believe that four hours had passed. I looked at my clock to make sure – 3:30 a.m. The last four hours were a blank space, completely unfelt, unlived, undreamt. This really was strong stuff.

I wasn't looking forward to my second dose. The thought of the flavor gave me the heebie-jeebies. Having no choice, I closed my eyes and drank it in one gulp. My body's natural reflexes urged me to throw it up, but I resisted the temptation, knowing that I needed this medication to walk.

Taylor reset our alarms for four hours later, 7:30 a.m., and climbed back over me to the other side of the bed. I put the second empty orange bottle on my filing cabinet and returned to sleep, falling into the unknown darkness of my new nighttime elixir.

Taylor woke up to our alarms at 7:30 a.m. and climbed over me to turn them off. We both needed to get to class, so he shook me awake. Hearing his voice over me, I mumbled, "Okay, I'm awake." Once again, the four hours had disappeared in a wink of the eye.

When I opened my eyes, fluorescent white light flooded in and my brain clenched up in violent pain. I closed them again, hoping the sensation would go away.

Taylor went to the bathroom to take a shower, leaving me lying in bed with a pulsating headache and closed eyes. I promptly fell back asleep until he re-awoke me when he returned from the shower. My headache was even worse when I stood up, but I was late for class.

"Come on, Julie," I whispered to myself, as if psyching myself up for a tough squash match. I proceeded to the bathroom to get ready for the day.

Elise knew I had started my new nighttime medication the night before and emailed me in the morning. "How are you feeling?" I didn't want to complain but she asked, so I told her the truth. The headache stayed strong all day. I went through the motions at school, but was greatly distracted by the pressure in my brain. I blamed the medication and dreaded having to take it again that night.

The next couple of days, I woke up with headaches of varying degrees. Some mornings, I also had a stomach ache and nausea, and was unable to look at food for hours, even though my stomach grumbled loudly. Elise continued to email me regularly to check in. I appreciated being able to vent.

One afternoon, a particularly strong headache took command of my entire day. I sat in Intellectual Property class, trying to take notes. My vision went blurry. I stopped typing notes and lifted my hands to my face to massage my temples. It seemed that the ceiling of the room was caving in and the weight of the floors above – all five stories of bricks and cement was sitting directly on top of my skull.

I left class to go to the bathroom, certain I would throw up. Standing over a toilet, I gagged and spit up saliva for a few minutes. My eyes watered from the gagging. The pressure remained. I cleaned up at the sink, wiping my eyes dry, before robotically returning to the classroom.

After class, I darted for the parking lot to drive home. Not far from my apartment, I got stuck in a traffic jam for a Red Sox game. Unable to take the throbbing pain anymore, I pulled over by the Museum of Fine Arts, less than a minute from my apartment, parked in the first spot I could find, and fell asleep. When I awoke half an hour later, my head felt much better, as if someone had untied the terrible knots in my brain while I slept.

Later that afternoon, back in my apartment, I called the Xyrem specialty pharmacy to inquire about the side effect of bad headaches. The pharmacist said that they didn't have any information on splitting headaches as a major side effect from the medication, which surprised me, as I was certain my reoccurring headaches were a result of taking the drug.

Although sick in new ways, Xyrem was improving my cataplexy tremendously. Dr. Larson had said it would take a few weeks before I would feel the full effects, I noticed an improvement right away. I could laugh and feel emotions without the physical weakness snatching my entire body away. My love life improved immediately – sexual excitement no longer paralyzed me.

Sometimes, usually late at night, the same emotional triggers sent a tingling sensation to my head and crossed over into muscle weakness. My knees still gave out on me and I lost my grip on a cup occasionally, but these were much more manageable moments of weakness. The Xyrem had brought me up off the ground.

Yet it couldn't erase my fresh memories of more extreme cataplexy attacks. The times I'd collapsed to the ground before starting Xyrem still hung heavy in my mind. I'd hoped to sweep these experiences under the rug, pretend I'd never known the powerlessness of my muted body, but those moments that once lived in my bones and muscles, were unforgettable.

Subsequently, small moments of cataplexy were laced with a much larger fear – a fear of falling. Even a small buckle of the knees made me anxious, knowing the possibility of full collapse. Once I lost trust in my body supporting me, it was hard to regain that faith. The small episodes of cataplexy were stinging reminders of the bigger disconnect that had grown between me and my body.

While I was adjusting to all this, law school life continued on, full speed ahead, and I tried to keep up, refusing to let narcolepsy get in the way. In mid-October, I returned home from a softball game and checked the mailbox on my way upstairs.

A thin envelope from my old law firm sat on top. My hands trembled as I ripped it open and unfolded the single piece of paper. The letter, on familiar letterhead was addressed to "Ms. Flygare," and was only three sentences long. There was no sugar coating it – I hadn't gotten the job.

I stuffed the news back in the envelope and continued upstairs slowly, eyes wide with shock. Admittedly, my chances had been slim, given my first year grades, yet some small pathetic part of me had held out hope, probably because I had no other plan – no alternative dream to fall back on.

ELEVEN
MONSTER

THE APARTMENT WAS HOT – the good kind of hot, but hot none-the-less, simmering with anticipation and fun. Fall was my favorite season. This was Halloween night and Tracy and I were about to host a pre-party before the law school's official Halloween bash.

I stood over a steamy stovetop, mulling hot cider with cinnamon sticks and rum. Tracy sat at the kitchen table, frosting pumpkin-shaped sugar cookies. Taylor zipped around the apartment hanging black and orange streamers and life-size skeleton cut outs. Tracy and I were a good party hosting team and Taylor enjoyed helping.

The air was thick with cinnamon and sugar. Everyone commented on how good it smelled as they entered. Costumes flooded in and the temperature kept rising. We opened the big bay windows to the crisp autumn air, but it was of little help as our cozy apartment spilled over cozy capacity.

Five, then 10, then 25 of our friends arrived. Beads of sweat gathered under my bangs as I ladled spiked cider into mugs.

I wasn't wearing my costume yet, opting to stay in my gym shorts and t-shirt to wait out the heat wave. Plus, I was concerned with getting my guests their drinks. We had a variety of high end pumpkin-laced and Oktoberfest-themed beers in the fridge. Weaving between friends and furniture, I passed out cold beer and hot cider. The cider was a hit, and I rushed back to the kitchen to start up a second batch.

Our apartment quickly turned to chaos, but I loved it like this, so alive and spirited. In the kitchen and living room, people in costumes mingled amongst one another, eating chips and salsa, drinking and posing for pictures. In the bathroom and hallway, those with incomplete costumes attended to last minute details and alterations, safety pins, makeup, and glitter hairspray. It was a theater's dressing room on opening night.

One friend graciously accepted my offer of hot cider, but asked, "Where's your drink?"

I looked him over. He held his Nixon mask in one hand and the cider in the other. A hint of whiskey surfaced between us. He must have pre-pre-partied before the pre-party.

"Oh, I don't drink anymore," I scooted past him, hoping to leave it at that, but glanced back and noticed his bewildered expression. He looked like I'd just told him I sold my soul to the devil.

It was getting late, I thought I'd better put on my costume. My bedroom was much cooler. I shut the door behind me and breathed a big sigh of relief.

The costume email chain had started weeks ago between my law school girlfriends. Ideas were gathered and thrown around, until we eventually decided to go as a Miss America competition. Tracy would be Miss South Carolina, and I'd dress as Miss Puerto Rico. We'd also have Miss Alaska, Miss Nevada, Miss California, Miss Florida, Miss Texas, Miss Louisiana, and Miss West Virginia.

Miss Nevada hosted a sash designing party where we used ribbons, glitter glue and puffy paints to design sashes with our respective state names.

Some females use Halloween as an excuse to wear skimpy revealing clothing, but I was never one of those girls. Dressing up as Miss Puerto Rico, I'd purchased a floor length flamenco dancer style dress; iridescent pearl white fabric with pink and teal accents and frills. The skirt puffed out considerably, with seven layers of stiff hot fabric.

The outfit came with a matching head piece, a white turban filled with plastic fruit – bright purple grapes, an apple and a few bananas, all dipped in a vat of glitter. I'm not sure why I thought this get up looked Puerto Rican, but I went with it anyway.

Looking back, I can see the whole night, from beginning to end, from two very different points-of-view: the night I wanted it to be and the night that it was. I wish I could say that it started out well and turned sour later on, but in reality, it was terrible from the beginning.

I'd been taking Xyrem for over a month now and although it was drastically improving my cataplexy, I was still waking up with pounding headaches some mornings. Halloween was one of those days. My senses were heightened so everything around me sent daggers of pain from one side of my head to the other – bright lights, loud voices, and hot bodies. I usually loved all this; hosting parties was my specialty, but tonight, it was my personal hell.

While our guests milled around the rest of the apartment, I stood in my room, looking at my costume resting peacefully across my bed. Some pieces were homemade and I'd bought others online. It had taken strategic planning to pull it all together, but now I wanted to lie down next to it and call it a night. My eyes burned so forcefully I could almost hear the pain, like the sizzling of a branding iron. It was hard to think. I was sure going to bed would make it stop.

As a "good sleeper" most of my life, I'd grown to rely on this easy escape. If I didn't want to deal with a particular feeling or moment – mostly boring car rides or depressing nights alone – I slept it off. I lost many other moments to sleep too, moments I didn't want to lose, so it wasn't always a solace, but a bad headache was one of the things I could easily pass over with a nap in the past.

I told myself everyone has days like this, when Advil doesn't do the trick, when pain turns to nausea because there's nowhere else for it to go. The only solution I'd found for this kind of day was to simply end the day by going to sleep.

Knock, knock.

"Who is it?"

Taylor poked his head in, entered and shut the door behind him. He turned to check himself out in the full-length mirror behind my door. He was particularly proud of his racecar driver costume – helmet, jumpsuit and all. He even had a fake steering wheel to "steer" his way around. He was anxious for some photos of his costume, so I took a series of solo shots for him to share with his friends and family. He wasn't usually into photos, so his enthusiasm was dorky and endearing.

When satisfied with his photo shoot, Taylor looked me over in my gym clothes. "What are you doing? Get into your costume already!"

"I know, I know. It's just that my head hurts."

I'd already told him about my headache, but couldn't help repeating myself. It was all I could think about. He didn't say anything as we stood there staring at each other, the noise of the party reverberating against my bedroom door.

"I don't want to go back out there."

Taylor continued to look at me. "Why not?"

"I don't know. I just can't handle it right now."

There was another awkward moment before he spoke. "I don't see why this is so difficult, Julie. It's all of *your* best friends out there."

Taylor rarely expressed frustration toward me, yet this statement was soaked in anger. He may as well have spit on me, and worse, I felt that I deserved it.

My stomach dropped. He was right. I knew exactly who was out there. If

I listened closely, I could put a name to each and every voice on the other side of my bedroom door. These were the same voices that usually lifted my spirits, made me laugh, and gave me comfort.

The closer I listened, the more a repulsion grew in me, a repulsion for it all: the drinking, the energy, the costumes, and yes, all of *my* best friends. I wanted to disappear.

Only six weeks earlier, these same friends had given me a flashy feathered birthday tiara and danced the night away, bought me drinks, and showered me with love and attention. Now, their energy poured in through the crack at the bottom of the door like a blinding white light, and my brow furrowed in repugnance.

I wanted to be the life of the party. Like Taylor said, these were my best friends. What was so hard about it? The difficulty was in my head. Not on my face or seen in my eyes. It was deeper than that, under it all.

It wasn't a good feeling and I'm not proud of it. What kind of a monster invites friends over only to hide from them, sickened by their very presence? *I've lost my mind*, I thought, as I lifted the bottom of my t-shirt up to begin changing.

Taylor left me to get ready on my own, perhaps trying to lead by example, to show me that my own party shouldn't be something to avoid. Soon, I could hear his voice through the door, chatting with a few of my friends.

He was not anti-social by any means, but I was usually the one who was more into this kind of thing. Taylor was on the quieter side around my friends, standing slightly behind me, interjecting funny comments here and there, but letting me carry the bulk of the small talk. These weren't his friends, they were my friends who knew Taylor as my boyfriend, but he faced them now with ease. He didn't need me there to help him with conversation. He was genuinely enjoying himself, I could tell because he talked a bit louder when excited – his voice coming from a deeper place inside himself.

Looking at my costume lying limp across my bedspread, I couldn't help but envy it. I would have given anything to let my costume go out for the night without me, leaving me to lie down in bed. But my immediate feelings and needs were of little importance in the big picture. I had to stuff the monster in the closet. There was no way around this night.

Delicately lifting the skirt up off my bed, I wrapped the seven layers of starched white fabric around my weary legs and placed the hat of fake apples, bananas and grapes onto my head. Thank goodness the glittery fruit was hollow – a turban of real fruit would have weighed heavily on my broken brain. I spread foundation over my entire face, highlighted my cheeks with bright blush and dazzled my eyelids with sparkles and mascara.

From under the fruit basket and behind the makeup, no one would be able to see the waves of stunted life, the restlessness and agitation gnawing at my head from the inside out. They would see what they wanted to see, and what I wanted them to see, the ruffles and glitter – the tacky and flashy costume that hid my reality, my disinterest, my wavering strength, my desire to get under the covers and go to bed.

Once decked out in festive gear, I checked my appearance in the full-length mirror. Who was under the costume anyway? The fun-loving attention-seeking Julie or someone who needed the night off? That's all I needed, one night off from being who I was supposed to be. Just one night. The timing was off. Most nights I didn't need to be much of anything to anyone – most nights, I could drift away into my alternate world of sleep. Not tonight.

I turned the doorknob slowly and stepped back into the limelight.

Slipping past Taylor, I caught his eyes for a second, painted a half-smile over my mouth and looked down, in quiet concession of my bad attitude in the bedroom. He came over and held my arm.

"I'm going to meet up with some friends at a bar to show them my costume. They aren't going to the law school party."

"Okay. Meet you at the party?"

"Great!" He seemed so happy, the cutting tone he'd used in the bedroom magically vaporized into thin air. A camera flash lit up the living room.

"Oh wait, Taylor, let's get a picture of us together first."

I asked a friend to take a photograph of us in our costumes – Miss Puerto Rico and the racecar driver. It wasn't our most romantic couple shot – the green and yellow of his jumpsuit clashed with the purples, pinks and creams of my costume, but it was fun to share Halloween together. Taylor stayed a few more minutes to take pictures of me with my friends, then left to meet his friends.

I made my way into the kitchen to greet Sophie, who had arrived while I was changing in my bedroom. She was dressed as the singer Amy Wine-house. She'd done an incredible job with her costume, looking more like the crazy punk singer than my college best friend. Fake tattoos snaked around her arms, her hair was disheveled and frizzy and her exaggerated eye makeup bordered on raccoon-esque. Sophie's Halloween spirit quickly brought a smile to my face.

"I haven't seen you in so long!" Sophie said.

The last time was my birthday, on the boat cruise. We'd said cheers and leaned back together under the thunderous applause of planes landing at Logan.

She admired my costume and then asked, "You started new medication right? So, you are feeling better?"

I thought about the heated tension in my head and gave an ambiguous shrug of the shoulders.

"Not really." I turned away from her to wash a mug and she leaned into the counter to face me.

"What's wrong, Julie?"

I swiveled a sponge along the inside of the mug, cleaning the cider from it. The neckline of my costume itched along the seam. "Nothing. Never mind." The kitchen was closing in on me. Sophie stared at me, waiting for more.

"The medications are making me feel like shit, okay?" My voice carried the vindictive rage of a belligerent drunk. "And this isn't the time or place to talk about it." I added with a snap.

"But I'm just asking." Sophie was zoned in. The party had fallen away from her mind. She had this incredible way of surrendering her full attention to the conversation at hand. It was one of her most endearing qualities, but in this instance, this same quality was suffocating me. She wanted to have this conversation right then, right there, not realizing that for me, the room was spinning madly around us. The noise and people were churning endlessly like a spitfire grill in my head. I couldn't afford to start talking about my medications at this point. Even the thought brought a threatening layer of wetness to my eyes. I was wearing too much makeup to let tears fall now and certainly didn't want to share my sadness with the 25 friends standing close by, as eager witnesses.

I swirled clean water around in the mug with tornado speed and turned the cup over, watching the water drip effortlessly from the mug's rim. Sophie was still standing there, saying nothing. *Why won't she just leave me alone,* I wondered.

"Not now, Sophie." I said, venom foaming at my lips.

I turned away from her once again, dropping the mug into the drying rack, and quickly exiting from the kitchen. I walked into the living room to greet other friends. Parties are meant to be blanketed in small talk, sprinkled with jokes and polite laughs. Deeper conversations, touching the monster under the mask, these are meant for late night car rides or desperate sobbing confessionals – one-on-one moments when you bare your ugliest self to another and hope they will still love you the next day.

Out of the corner of my eye, I watched Sophie slink out of the kitchen and join another group of friends in the living room. My stomach flipped. Did I really just storm off in the middle of our conversation?

Perhaps what angered me most about my discussion with Sophie was that she assumed that the medications would make me feel better. Unbeknownst to both of us, her question touched on the rawest of nerves inside me. A few months earlier, I'd assumed the same – that the medication would solve everything – piece of cake, end of story. Although I took my anger out on Sophie, I was truly mad at myself. What a fool I'd been.

"Julie?" Miss Alaska reached out to link around my waist. Another friend held a camera up, ready to capture the glam and glitter of our costumes.

"Right, sorry." I shuffled over to line up with the other pageanteers, flashing white teeth and big brown steady eyes, just in time to catch the lightening flash of the camera's shutter.

Around 9:30 p.m., we left for to the law school Halloween party at a bar a few blocks away. Inside the dark basement bar, I found Taylor, talking with a few softball friends. I ordered a Diet Coke and greeted the couple he was speaking with, dressed as Superman and Wonder Woman.

A little later, I joined my girlfriends on the dance floor to bop around to Kanye West's "Gold Digger." Sophie danced in this group, but I didn't try to make eye contact or dance next to her. I steered clear of her on purpose, petrified that she would be mad at me. I was ashamed, yet my lights were still dim. I was still looking through a lens of painful head pounding and didn't have the energy to try and make things right with Sophie that night.

Strangely, my exhaustion and pain shifted while I was on the dance floor, perhaps reaching a new state of exhaustion. My boundaries and inhibitions were broken down, I was energized by a sense of crazy lunacy. I began to genuinely enjoy myself, although the headache was still there. I transcended it for a few songs, concentrating on the music instead of my own body. I loved dancing and the DJ was playing some of my favorite artists, like Britney Spears and Jay-Z.

Couples started trickling out early, including Superman and Wonder Woman, who came over to say goodnight around 11:30 p.m. I envied them, but I didn't feel that I had the same freedom to just leave whenever I wanted to. Invisible strings attached me to the four corners of the room, strings of reliability, habit and friendship I wouldn't dare cut.

Some of my friends were getting pretty drunk. Miss Alaska and I nearly bumped into each other and I stopped, expecting we'd greet one another. She kept on walking, not noticing me and grabbed the arm of a guy in an orange prison jumpsuit. She was on the prowl for a new guy, which made me laugh. I loved silly nights like this, but I was not used to watching them as a sober outsider. Once I decided no one necessarily "needed" me anymore at the party, the strings attaching me to the room quickly unraveled. I was free to go home.

A few minutes past midnight, Taylor and I walked out of the dingy basement bar and back into the crisp New England night, heading back to my apartment. I'd never known what it was like to leave a party early. I felt a little guilty, but once outside, I let it go.

The walk home was the same few blocks we'd walked together on the night of our first date last January, almost 10 months earlier. We passed dark Fenway Park and I leaned against Taylor's chest. I fit there comfortably as ever.

Despite the drama between us of breaking up over the summer, we were still two pieces of the same puzzle. This was how things were meant to be. I breathed in the cold autumn air, sending a crackling chill up my spine.

"I love you," I said quietly.

"I love you too."

I hoped Taylor would forget my ugly words from earlier. Saying I didn't want to go out with my friends felt like treason. Instead of apologizing for earlier though, I said, "What a fun night!"

"Mhm." Taylor's voice hinted at an "I told you so." He didn't need to say it out loud. It was an obvious "win" for him and I didn't mind admitting my defeat in the subtlest of ways.

Social occasions were my bread and butter. Of course I'd had fun, but what made me happiest on the walk home wasn't how much fun I'd had, but how proud I was of myself that I'd survived. I was exhausted yet my spirit stood tall with pride.

It was strange to think of a social occasion as something to survive rather than somewhere to thrive, but tonight was an exception. It was bad timing with the massive headache and Halloween falling on the same day.

A misty rain slowly sifted through the dark night sky. I took off my shoes and walked the last two blocks barefoot, lifting my iridescent pearl, seven layer skirt slightly off the damp pavement. The refreshing air was like extra oxygen, loosening the balls of tightness in my head. Sure, the evening started out roughly, but I rebounded nicely.

Once home, I hurried to the bathroom to mix my nighttime medication, wipe my face clear of the caked makeup and glitter, and brush my teeth.

In my bedroom, I looked at my bed with excitement bubbling in my chest. An internal voice said, "This bed is your prize for being so good tonight. You can lie down now, wash away into nothingness and stay there as long as your little heart desires."

I unzipped the costume, let the stiff layers of fabric fall to the floor, and climbed into bed in just my underwear. Like finally giving into a sexual attraction with someone that has built up over time, finally allowing my body to touch my sheets and pillows was a cherished moment of pure joy. It was the moment I'd yearned for all day and imagined over and over like an unattainable fantasy. It was the moment that had clouded my judgment and stolen my attention away from many other moments.

Eyes half shut, I reached over to my side table and eagerly gulped down my first nasty dose of Xyrem. My alarm was set to take my second dose at 5 a.m. I turned away from the medicine, letting the soft white sheets envelope my weary skin. A few seconds later, Taylor gingerly climbed over me to the other side of my bed. *I couldn't be any more content*, I thought, as I disappeared.

Taylor woke me at 5 a.m. for my second dose. When I woke again around 10 a.m., my head was still inside the sleep vacuum. I returned to sleep's doorstep on hands and knees, begging to be let back in. Sleep opened the door and let me free fall back in. It could steal as much of my Sunday as it wanted.

Of course there were other things I could have done, like homework or exercise – but I didn't feel too guilty. Taylor was tired and slept in, too. Talking with friends later in the afternoon, I learned that they also slept in, hung over from the festivities the night before. Even though I hadn't had any alcohol on Halloween, when I finally got out of bed around 1 p.m. on Sunday, my head was ringing with anger as if I'd had too much to drink.

Experiencing the familiar depletion of life that I used to feel after a big night out drinking didn't seem fair. Perhaps the exertion of hosting the pre-party and going out until midnight put me over the edge. Things were changing.

TWELVE
PROMISES

AFTER HALLOWEEN, friction grew between Taylor and I. While driving to the library one day, I spoke with him on the phone. I'd just been to the gym and was tired from my physical therapy exercises and light workout. I had a lot of homework to do. Exercising used to be a stress-relieving, energizing part of my day. Now it left me in a haze.

"I'm not sure I can exercise and study on the same day anymore. I don't have the energy for both."

Taylor was silent.

"It's frustrating, you know?"

"Yeah." He didn't seem to get it so I tried a different angle.

"What if you weren't able to workout because of an illness? Would that upset you?"

"Yeah, I'm sure, Julie." He worked out regularly, his physique meant a lot to him, but he didn't seem to be sympathizing.

Perhaps I shouldn't have been surprised that Taylor and I struggled to connect about my narcolepsy. He hadn't been able to empathize with my feelings the summer before.

In another conversation, he told me that he felt awkward drinking around me now. Not drinking alcohol made me self-conscious, but I tried to be upbeat while socializing at bars. I even bought drinks for friends occasionally to show I was still "fun" and wanted them to drink around me. Hearing that my non-drinking was hindering Taylor's happiness only doubled my shame.

Despite Taylor's lack of understanding, I clung to our relationship tighter than ever. My self-confidence reached an all time low. I believed I was lucky to have Taylor – he knew my old self, the person I wanted to be. I feared that no one could ever possibly love me like this.

A week after Halloween, we were walking down the stairs to leave his apartment when a wave of dread came over me. I stopped half way down the stairwell.

"Do you love me?"

"Of course." He placed his hands on my shoulders, stopping short behind me on the stairs.

"Yeah, okay." My stomach was uneasy. "But do you *really* love me?"

"Yes. Why?" It wasn't like me to question his affection. Tears welled in my eyes. "I dunno. I'm just afraid."

"Afraid of what?"

"Afraid of loving you."

He drew his head back like a turtle, surprised and unsure of where this was coming from.

"I'm scared because I think I'm falling even deeper for you, like I really *really* love you in a big uncontrollable way."

"Okay." He was always so even-tempered.

"But what if you don't love me back like that?" Tears streamed down my face. Taylor rubbed my back as I cried. My emotions were fragile – resting in his hands.

"What do you think?"

"I think you have to just let go, Julie."

"What do you mean?" I tried to breathe slowly to stop crying.

"You can't control your feelings. Sure, love is scary, but you just have to let go and fall. You can't be so afraid of what will come of it."

It wasn't the answer I'd been looking for. I was hoping he would say I had nothing to worry about because he'd be by my side forever. Yet his perspective on opening one's heart to love was perhaps the most self-reflective comment Taylor had ever made. Maybe we were connecting on a more personal "deep" level, finally. I regained my composure and we continued on our way, though my fears soon resurfaced.

Taylor started going out more often with his friends without me. I was happy to let him go out while I stayed home and relaxed. The bar scene was losing its appeal for me anyway, and I'd never been jealous before, but I started asking him about his female friends and checked Facebook.com for any photos of him with other women. Perhaps my behavior was crazy, or maybe I intuitively sensed that he was drifting from me.

About two weeks after Halloween, things fell apart. I texted Taylor one evening to ask when he was coming to sleep over. He was out at a bar with his friends near my apartment. He texted back saying he was going to share a cab with friends and sleep at home, alone. My apartment was much closer. It didn't make sense. We spent almost every night together. My heart raced. I texted back asking what was going on. He didn't respond. I called and left a voicemail, but got no response.

After a restless night, I woke up to a cold, rainy day in Boston, still without a word from Taylor. I called Dad.

"Good morning, Jules. What's up?"

"Taylor is acting strange. I'm afraid I may lose him."

"Why would you think that?"

I explained how I'd been so insecure, questioning Taylor about his female friends and worrying I loved him more than he loved me.

"Relationships are like that. Sometimes one person relies heavily on the other, but it goes back and forth. That's the beauty of relationships."

This was reassuring. I certainly hadn't always been so needy. It was a temporary phase. I was adjusting to narcolepsy.

"But he was out with his friends last night and ignored my text and phone call. He's never done that!"

"You're drawing conclusions quickly, Jules. He loves you – he'll work to make things right."

I was so grateful I could rely on Dad to talk me down from my dramatic, irrational moments. We discussed the possibility that my medications were to blame. Dr. Larson had warned me that depression could be an issue with Xyrem. I wasn't sure this was depression, but I wasn't feeling like myself. Dad suggested I call Dr. Larson's office to look into it.

He also encouraged me to write Taylor an email saying that I was looking into changing my medicines because I was afraid they were making me unstable and suggesting we should spend some time apart while I worked it out. I sent the email right away.

Taylor emailed back, saying he had class at 10 a.m., then he was going to the gym. He wanted to stop by around 1 p.m. to talk.

I was nervous all morning, unable to concentrate on my schoolwork. I tried repeating Dad's comforting advice in my head, but still feared Taylor would break up with me.

Before 1 p.m., I gathered the things Taylor kept in my apartment into a paper bag. In case he broke up with me, I'd be ready. I hid the bag in the front hall closet. When Taylor arrived I let him in, then sat cross-legged on my bed while he stood in the middle of my bedroom, his gray workout clothes wet with sweat and fresh raindrops.

Still out of breathe from the stairs, he dived right in, "I think we should break up." The room was dead silent. It was my worst nightmare.

"Any reason?" my voice quivered.

"I can't give you an exact reason." He spoke quickly and in a matter-of-fact tone. "I just know that I've checked out of this relationship, and I know myself. Once I'm checked out, I'm not going to come back. Taking a break won't work. It's over."

I bit my bottom lip.

He probably thought it was honorable to do this in person, but it didn't feel like "in person" to me since the person standing before me wasn't the Taylor I'd known and loved.

"Okay, I want to say that I love you, and I'm sorry it didn't work out between us. I'm glad we gave it a second try, though."

He stared blankly.

"So, you can't give me any reason?"

"No, not right now."

"I have your stuff packed."

"Oh, I didn't bring yours." This was the first hint of softness in his voice.

"That's okay." I felt a small sense of pride in having prepared the bag. He'd broken my heart, but he hadn't caught me off guard.

This small victory created a tingling in my head, the warning signal of cataplexy. If I hadn't been on Xyrem, I most likely would have collapsed. Yet I climbed off my bed, walked feebly to the closet without any external weakness showing and handed Taylor the bag at the door.

He turned and left without looking back.

I shut the door and ran to my bed and cried. Within minutes, I called

Dad and told him Taylor had broken up with me.

"I'll be there as soon as I can. Will you be all right until I get there?"

"Yeah."

Within an hour and a half, Dad was outside my apartment, waiting in his old silver Volvo. I hurried to his car through a downpour of rain carrying a small overnight bag of essentials.

Once in the safety of Dad's presence, I reclined my seat and sobbed violently during the ride home to New Hampshire. He stayed quiet and kept his eyes on the road ahead, letting me cry out my pain without interruption. Throughout the years, during my worst moments of despair, he had come to save me like this, whisking me away from my greatest disappointments, shattered relationships mostly.

At Dad and Diana's house, I spent an embarrassing amount of time clenched up in a ball and slouched over, constantly in motion, trying to dislodge the hurt. It was no use.

Taylor had betrayed my trust. My heart was broken. Yet strangely, something else came to the surface as hurting more – narcolepsy. I had tried to ignore it by concentrating on my relationship but now, with no relationship, I faced this deeper source of hurt and uncertainty.

If Taylor didn't love me, who else would? He'd known and loved me before narcolepsy. It was my only hope. Now that I took medication twice a night and didn't have the energy to go out to bars on weekends, how would I meet someone? How would I explain this insanity? I had so many unanswered questions about how dating could ever be normal with all the recent changes. I'd been diagnosed and taking the best treatment options for two months, but things were not resolved as I'd expected.

I finally lay still on the floor of Dad and Diana's bedroom. Dad sat on the edge of his bed, watching me drown in my sadness.

The prickly carpet itched my hot skin. I closed my bloodshot eyes and concentrated on the darkness within. Inside this lonesome interior, I felt as if thick leather straps were constricting around my body, crushing me, until I had no strength left.

I wished that the carpet would open and take me. I imagined falling out of this existence – the release, the bliss. *If only I could lose myself. If only I could disappear*, I thought.

Eyes still closed, I broke the silence, "Narcolepsy is the worst thing that's ever happened to me. I hate it so much, I want to crush it."

Dad didn't respond. I wasn't necessarily speaking *to* him anyway. I was just speaking and he was just there, listening.

"Eventually, I'm going to make narcolepsy the *best* thing that ever happened to me. I'm going to turn it on its head."

Still no response from Dad. My own voice echoed over and over in my head. I wanted revenge on narcolepsy. I had to believe I could overcome it in some way. Although I had no idea how I would do this, the promise stuck with me.

The diagnosis and medication process was deceiving. Everything moved forward so quickly, it seemed that "feeling better" was right around the corner. Thankfully, I'd left emotional collapsing in the dust where it belonged. I would go on with law school and life as planned. All this was just a speed bump.

Everyone assumed, like me, that this sickness was resolving itself. Naturally, no one sent me get well cards or flowers. I'd be better before I knew it. Or so it seemed.

THIRTEEN
A LION'S ROAR

L ATE ONE NIGHT, a week after the breakup, I saw Taylor at school and our eyes locked. I was on my way to my car and he was sitting in the Yellow Room, typing on his laptop, which was strange since he never studied at school.

I smiled and lifted my hand to wave. Instinctively, my body leaned in his direction, then quickly stopped. His mouth rose slightly, as if acknowledging a street beggar.

The tingling aura flowed through my head. The closest objects were the chairs at Taylor's table 15 feet away or, if I turned around, the doorway 10 feet behind me. The Yellow Room presented a particularly challenging place for my cataplexy. Making it from one side to the other took concentration and luck. If I fell, I fell before an audience. Friends presented a risk – seeing a friend might make me laugh, which would be dangerous. Seeing my ex-boyfriend was a new risk.

I re-focused on the ground to clear my mind. Miraculously, my knees caught themselves as they should. I put one foot in front of the other – moving steadily.

This was the magic of the Xyrem – holding my body up when I felt emotions, an invaluable benefit making the nausea and headaches worthwhile. A few months before, this moment would have almost certainly buckled my knees and perhaps lead to collapse in public. Now, I moved forward like a product on a conveyor belt – past Taylor and out of the Yellow Room.

I stood in the parking lot with my heart pounding and jitters climbing up my throat. It was too awful. Surely he'd follow me. He'd come for me any second now.

I cupped my face in my hands and sobbed. He wasn't chasing me. I continued on to my car. Driving home, my mind raced. How could he treat me like this? What had I done? Who was this rude stranger?

At a red light at the intersection where I used to turn off to go to Taylor's apartment, my fingers gripped the steering wheel tightly. When the light turned green, I pressed the gas hard and jerked myself back into motion along the deserted four-lane road toward Fenway.

I inhaled but my lungs only filled with toxic anger. I don't know where the fire began, or how it spread so ferociously, but when I breathed out, flames emerged from the pit of my stomach.

My mouth opened and a violent loud "WHY?" filled the car.

When out of breath, I inhaled quietly, unsure about what just happened. I'd never heard anything like it – certainly not from my own body. I slowed down and drove the speed limit. The scream had startled me.

My mouth opened wide and again, a lion's roar came out.

I hated loud noises, yet an ear-piercing scream from within emerged again and again. I couldn't stop. It was shameful, but no one would have to know, since my rage was muffled behind the tightly sealed doors and windows of my car.

My throat burned, as if real flames incinerated my insides.

Reaching the Charles River, I hugged a right turn for the final stretch of the drive. Usually the view of the river reflecting the sparkling light of the skyscrapers soothed me, but tonight I was too shaken to enjoy it.

Entering my neighborhood, the matching red brick buildings with bay windows, the old-fashioned street lanterns and picket fences enclosing manicured lawns all struck me as clean and neat. Everything fit within the lines here, it was all cookie-cutter and perfect. Pleasantville. Tonight, I didn't belong here.

A pedestrian passed in front of my car. Although I was pretty sure she wouldn't be able to hear, I stopped screaming just in case.

I was possessed by a malevolent spirit and didn't recognize this self, a person with a terrifying rage I'd never known.

Opening my car door, I returned to myself, the one living in Pleasantville. I felt strangely better. I opened the apartment door quietly, and tiptoed to my bedroom, being careful not to disturb Tracy, asleep in her room.

I mixed my Xyrem in the bathroom and counted the hours to figure out when I had to get up for the second dose. I set multiple alarms, knowing I might not wake up to any of them and miss my window of opportunity to take my second dose. This had been much easier with Taylor's help.

One night at the library, I glanced down at my phone, hoping Taylor would call or text, though I hadn't heard from him since he ended things, nor had I tried contacting him. I envisioned him calling or emailing or texting to apologize and ask for me back. I had so much to say to him, how could he have nothing to tell me? It took Herculean patience to resist contacting him, but I held off. When he wanted me, he'd contact me. So I waited.

I did have a new voicemail from my stepmother, Diana.

"It's about Dad, call me back."

Phone calls were not allowed in the library, so I rushed downstairs to the atrium outside the library and dialed Diana's cell phone. No answer. It was almost 9 p.m. She usually never called so late.

Unable to reach her, I started to call Dad directly but hesitated. I called my sister instead.

"Things aren't looking good," she said. "He received some bad test results."

"What do you mean by bad?" I talked loudly. A few students were studying in the atrium, but I didn't care. My body boiled. I'd just seen him. How could this be happening?

Dad had a weak heart. Two years earlier, he had an operation to implant a pacemaker and defibrillator. Soon after, he had a minor stroke. After each bad incident, I lived in fear of the next urgent call for a while, then slowly got over it, only to receive a call when I least expected it.

"He may be a candidate for a heart transplant," my sister explained.

A heart transplant had been mentioned before as a distant possibility, in hushed voices when Dad wasn't in the room. Our fear, it seemed, was now coming true. My hero was an older man with human restrictions, made of flesh and blood and 100 percent breakable. Over the next few days, I talked about the heart transplant with Diana, my sister, my brother and eventually Dad.

I conducted these conversations from the atrium outside the library, when I was supposed to be studying for finals. I was scared and couldn't believe this was happening now. In addition to narcolepsy, the breakup, the job rejection, and exams approaching, this was much too much. It felt like an out of body experience. Actually, Dad's health problems helped put the breakup into perspective. How could I cry about stupid Taylor when I could lose my hero?

All I could do was wait and continue with my life at school. I stayed studying late every night. It was hard to concentrate and sleepiness came often.

One night, while studying at a group table in the library, I looked at the clock to see it was past 9 p.m., and realized that I hadn't taken a nap yet. Usually by this hour, my daytime stimulant, Provigil, had worn off and I'd already thrashed in and out of fogginess at least a few times, taking a nap or two or fighting off the excruciating heaviness.

This night, there was absolutely no heaviness pushing down on my skull, no clogged connections in my brain, no nagging at my eyelids. The feeling of *nothing* would usually go undetected, but it was so foreign to me that nothing seemed like *something*.

In the hushed silence of the law library, tears streamed down my cheeks and fell into the crease of my textbook. I didn't bother to hide my face or wipe my tears. Instead, I sat still, in awe of this strange self-realization.

The gap between wakefulness and sleepiness was much wider than I'd thought. I'd lost touch entirely with what true wakefulness felt like. I saw it now as powerful because it was so free, I could think and study and make connections without any heaviness on my head.

I decided that this was my nighttime medication, Xyrem, improving my wakefulness independently from the daytime stimulant, Provigil. On Provigil, all my sensations were heightened and I was amped up, which somewhat masked my sleepiness, but not entirely. I often felt both jittery and exhausted simultaneously.

This wakefulness was different, it was quiet and calm, as if someone lifted the weight off my skull and allowed my brain to work at its own pace. I savored the freedom inside my skull.

Later that night, I wandered to the café to take a break from studying and realized that I hadn't eaten yet. It hadn't occurred to me once all day, and I wasn't hungry, even now, past 11 p.m.

The café had many options – a grill, pasta bar, sandwich bar, sushi, salads, chips, cookies, hummus, pita and fruit. Each one made me more nauseated. I began panicking. I needed to eat something, but I'd never been so repulsed by food.

I settled on an English Muffin. I toasted the muffin, added peanut butter and jelly, and lifted it to my mouth.

I didn't want to eat it, but forced myself to take a bite. I closed my eyes, chewed and swallowed it down, with my head shaking in disgust.

It's PB&J, not poison.

I lifted the English Muffin to my mouth again. On my third bite, my eyes were wet with tears. I couldn't do it. I threw the remainder away and hurried back to the library.

I'd always been a good eater. I loved food. This wasn't me. The medications were part of the problem. Provigil wiped out my appetite during the day and Xyrem left me nauseated in the morning. I wasn't allowed to eat two hours before bedtime, and I wasn't hungry during the day. Now, with the breakup and Dad's health situation, my appetite had disappeared completely.

When I started the medications, I quickly lost the extra 15 pounds I'd never had before narcolepsy, but then, the weight loss kept going, and I reached an all-time low of 138, about 15 pounds lower than my normal weight, for a total loss of 30 pounds in five months. My jeans slipped on and off without unbuttoning them.

One of my best friends let me go through her old clothes. She had a few pairs of nice jeans that fit perfectly, which was a relief. Lying in bed some mornings, I touched my flat stomach, as if exploring unfamiliar territory. I liked my skinnier body, but it was foreign. I'd been on and off of diets since seventh grade, always struggling with my weight. Now, the one time I hadn't been trying, the pounds disappeared seemingly overnight – the product of sickness, sadness and nausea.

"Are you being healthy?" my brother asked. A few friends said that they were worried about me.

I'd gained 15 pounds in three months and no one said a thing. Now, I'd lost 30 pounds in five months and everyone was concerned. I looked good, but no, I wasn't healthy. I had an illness that was challenging me in new ways. I'd been struggling to communicate this to my loved ones. It wasn't until my outer appearance changed that others became worried.

I screamed in my car almost every night now. It became a habit I didn't like, but I couldn't stop myself. I didn't tell anyone – it was my little secret.

Maybe it was the jealousy and passion of my failed romance. Though I'd had other breakups, and various other disappointments and betrayals before, they'd never filled me with a lion's roar.

Returning home late one night, I found a large manila envelope on the kitchen table from the Narcolepsy Network, the narcolepsy patient organization. I'd ordered a bunch of informational materials soon after my diagnosis – practically everything for sale on the site – CDs, tapes, pamphlets and a guide to understanding narcolepsy. I was so excited to learn more, but when? I saved it for the weekend.

That Friday night, I curled up with the materials as Tracy prepared to go out to a bar.

"Are you sure you don't want to join me?" she asked.

"Yes, thank you."

We used to go out together. Our weekends had consisted of going to softball and brunch by day and out to bars by night. Now, my body ached so much from weekday activities, I looked forward to resting on weekends and not having to rush my nighttime medication process.

I started reading the guide to understanding narcolepsy to learn more about the science behind the disorder and other patients' experiences with the symptoms and treatments.

It seemed that people with narcolepsy found social relations challenging. I'd been bewildered by the social distance I felt from my friends and guilty for ruining my relationship with Taylor. Maybe this was normal. Other people with narcolepsy reported not having as much energy as before. I'd been so mad at myself for not having my same high energy level.

The guide said that school and jobs could be challenging for people with narcolepsy, but I couldn't accept this for myself. I was going to be successful. Of course, having been rejected from my dream job at the firm, I didn't know what I'd do next, but once I made a new game plan, I'd succeed. Then, I could inspire others. Yes, that was what I would do.

I'd never met another person with narcolepsy. I'd only read about them and watched a few video interviews online. I was realizing that maybe narcolepsy wasn't the small illness I'd originally assumed it was. I thought I was going to take medication and feel better. The drugs had improved my symptoms, but hadn't erased them entirely. Plus, the side effects were strong and I would be taking these drugs for how long? Life? The materials validated my experience of this being a difficult disorder but in doing so, opened my eyes to the possibility that narcolepsy wasn't just going away.

The following Monday, I woke up out of the complete darkness of my nighttime medication with my head pulsating in pain and my stomach growling – all common side effects. I rolled over, placing my face in my pillow. I wanted to stay in bed, but I had to hurry to school for class. I was running late, something else that was becoming common. I drove down the four-lane road, sitting impatiently at the red light by the turn to Taylor's house, and thought back over the past couple of weeks. I hadn't heard a word from Taylor. I thought of the job rejection and Dad's health. I thought of narcolepsy – the joke of an illness that was dominating my life. How was everything going wrong all at once?

The prospect of Taylor dumping me had felt like Armageddon in my mind. I truly couldn't imagine losing him. And then I did.

I'd always feared getting sick with something serious, like cancer or being bound to a wheelchair for life. Narcolepsy wasn't cancer or a wheelchair, but I was realizing it was life changing. I'd feared losing Dad and that was becoming a possibility, too. I'd feared doing poorly in law school and not getting the big fancy job, which was also happening.

I'd spent an embarrassing portion of the last few weeks crying. I'd rolled around on the rug in Dad's bedroom hoping that the floor would open and take me in. I'd screamed in my car night after night. I'd struggled and I would struggle more, but all at once it hit me —my worst fears had come true. What else did I have to be afraid of now? No one could take anything else away from me. I'd reached my bottom and yet, I was alive and breathing. No one understood my narcolepsy, but so what? *Forget them. Fight for yourself,* I told myself. I was alone and everything had fallen to pieces. And now I was free.

The sun glistened through the trees as I continued driving toward law school. How beautiful, I thought. The sun was shining and I was breathing. This was enough. Maybe this was how dying people feel – they have nothing left to be scared of and they're set free.

Later that day at school, I decided to email Taylor. It had been almost a month. I knew his response would not be what I wanted, but my new sense of bravery pushed me onward. It was pathetic, but I didn't care.

In my email, I asked for a greater explanation. I said that I didn't understand and thought we shouldn't throw our relationship under the bus. I sat in my cubicle in the library basement, my heart pounding as I hit send.

He responded within the hour, explaining that we weren't having fun together, and that I'd see that with time. It was cold. This wasn't the person I'd loved. He was gone, and this time I believed him.

I had to return to studying since my exams were quickly approaching, but my head was on another planet now. I rushed out of the library, unsure of where to go. I could've gone home but it would be no different. There was no escaping this moment.

I walked to my car and sat in silence. The windows steamed up as I breathed heated sighs of sadness. Tears soon came. How could he be so cold to me? My hands gripped the seat cushion.

The view was desolate and dead – small groupings of trees and rocks, roots and mulch. There were no leaves on the trees, making the slumber of approaching winter all too apparent. After a few minutes, I still didn't feel like driving, so I called Dad.

"Apparently, we weren't having fun!" I gushed, "No kidding! I was dealing with a new illness. How could he be so heartless?"

"I don't know, Julie, it's weird."

Dad told me about a program he saw on TV about empathy – how when older couples had been together for 30 or 40 years and one person was in pain, the other literally felt it. Scientists had researched this and concluded it's the highest form of empathy, that two people are so bonded they can physically feel the other's pain.

"In contrast, teenage boys are on the end of the empathy scale," he explained. "Taylor is closer to that end."

I was captivated by Dad's insightful reflection, partly because his words were comforting, and also because it was cool to hear him reflect on emotions. The stoic man was opening up.

Sometimes I caught him when he was busy and although I knew he'd rather talk to me, he was usually in the middle of something – a meeting or driving to a meeting. Today, I had his full attention.

"I've been thinking of you these last couple days," he reflected, "They've put me on this new medication that's been making me sick."

My stomach clenched. I'd forgotten to ask how he was feeling. He faced much bigger problems than my silly boy drama.

"Jules, I see now what you were saying about medication that's supposed to make you feel better, making you worse in other ways."

"Yeah, I know." I couldn't help laughing. Dad and I were bonding over the grunt work inside prescription orange pill bottles. I never thought that this is what the big-time lawyer and his superstar law school daughter would have in common. We'd been brought down to size by malfunctioning body parts – his heart, my brain.

It was nice that Dad was trying to better understand me and the complex system of symptoms and side effects. I always thought that he understood me.

The conversation felt so precious. After being fearful about Dad's decline in health, I'd stopped fighting it. Whatever was going to be would be and there was nothing to do but enjoy the time we had together now. The urgency and freedom between us was palpable. When you have only the moment directly in front of you with someone you love, it's incredible how drama, complication, and pettiness melt away. There was clarity that day; that what was most important was love and connection *now*, because that was all we had.

In a wave of honesty, I said, "I hate it here, Dad."

"I know."

What? He knew? I had complained about law school on many occasions, but I'd thought everyone was miserable. This was the first time I really meant it, I was surprised to hear that Dad already knew, or maybe he didn't really get it.

"No, I *really* hate it."

He was silent. Maybe he was reverting back to his usual less talkative self.

"Do you want to take some time off?"

I was caught off guard. Dean Wilson had brought it up as an option once. I'd dismissed the idea very quickly then. Now, I gave it a second thought.

I was almost half way through law school. What would I do if I took a break? A few images rushed through my head – folding sweaters at the Gap, my friends graduating without me, sitting in a class with younger students. Part of me knew that if I left law school now, I might never come back.

Taking a leave of absence didn't guarantee happiness either. "Happiness" didn't even seem like an achievable goal anywhere. Law school wasn't the most pleasant environment to adjust to narcolepsy and avoid an ex-boyfriend, but maybe what I hated wasn't law school but life in general. My problems weren't going to go away, and neither would the debt I'd already incurred going through the first half of law school.

Besides, I'd never considered quitting anything. I'd never transferred from a school or given up on anything I said I would do. Quitting wasn't in my vocabulary, or Dad's. This was the first time we had discussed anything remotely similar to quitting.

After some thought, taking some time off didn't seem the best option. I told Dad my reasoning and he agreed. He'd encouraged me to go to law school, so it was hard to discuss. It was a major relief to open up about this.

The words "take some time off" didn't need to be spoken again. It was nice to have had them out there once.

"It's really hard now," he said, "but I know this will make for a greater life, Jules. You will rise above."

I agreed, timidly. I was incredibly far from a higher place or a greater life, but it was nice to have him believe in me so much.

Driving home, I was much more at peace. Dad's words, emotions, laughter, and even the pauses had been filled with love and acceptance.

I knew I'd never be alone in the biggest sense of the word. Even if he died the next day, he'd always love me. He saw the very best in me, and no one could take that away from me. That was love in its purest form – someone carrying me when I reached my lowest point. I was heartbroken and drowning and Dad tossed me over his shoulders. His heart was weaker than ever, yet he gave me all his strength to stand on. We moved slowly, Dad and I, out of the darkness of December.

FOURTEEN

THIS TOO SHALL PASS

IN EARLY JANUARY, Sophie coordinated a group of 10 girls to go to a charity benefit at an art gallery in South Boston. It was fun to get dressed up in a black sparkly dress and high heels to attend a posh event and dance with friends, but when the event ended at 11 p.m., I was relieved. Time to go home and turn into a pumpkin.

Some of the girls hailed cabs and others piled into my car. I'd drive them back to Sophie's and then head home. Driving on nights out was an exciting new luxury due to my sobriety.

Sophie mentioned something about a concert. A friend of her new boyfriend was playing in a band at the Middle East club in Central Square near her house.

"Want to go?" Sophie asked the car full of girls.

"Sure," the girls called out from the back. "Sounds good!"

I smiled to myself. My old self would be right there with them. 11 p.m.

on a Saturday night used to be "early." I'd never been to the Middle East before but heard it was a cool club. I hadn't met Sophie's new boyfriend, Todd, who would be there, yet exhaustion loomed large for Sunday just from being out this late.

"I'll drop you guys off," I said. I was happy to deliver them safely to the club and then go home to bed.

"You sure? It will be fun."

"Yes, I'm sure. It's late and parking is impossible in Central."

Central Square was bustling with cars, pedestrians, police, buses, and bar hoppers. We inched toward the club, singing along with the radio. It had been a great night. When we arrived, Sophie pointed to a parking space directly in front.

"Park here and come meet Todd. It won't take long."

I double-checked the signs to make sure the spot was legal. "Okay, but just for a few minutes."

The girls tumbled out of my car and into the club. I gripped the railing and stepped carefully in my high heels down the steep narrow staircase, to the concert downstairs. We were slightly overdressed, so heads turned as we entered the dark underground concert venue.

The club was an ordinary basement with lots of ordinary Boston guys wearing flannel shirts and Red Sox hats. For some reason, I'd pictured the Middle East as some sort of exotic international hip place. This was more like a sticky frat basement and not my scene, especially not while wearing a semi-formal dress.

Sophie found Todd right away.

"Nice to meet you," he said politely, then turned his full attention to Sophie, and grabbed her ravenously around the waist. He seemed pretty drunk. Sophie smiled sheepishly.

Some girls approached the crowded bar to get drinks. I went with them to get myself a Diet Coke and to give Sophie and Todd some alone time, then I joined the group on the dance floor, dancing and clapping. Each band performed only a few songs and I don't remember if we saw the band we had come to hear.

Our group broke apart quickly, with some girls sitting on bar stools complaining of sore feet and others leaving to find a bar with a more up-scale crowd. I had a second wind of energy and forgot about going home. By midnight, just Sophie, Todd and I remained on the dance floor, sand-wiched in a sea of strangers.

Sophie and Todd danced closely. Still in the honeymoon phase, they couldn't get enough of one another. Alcohol relaxed their bodies into each other. They showed affection outwardly – infatuation at its finest. It was endearing and sickening at the same time. They were drunk, I was sober. They were together, I was alone. This was a familiar scenario. I'd been the third wheel of Sophie's love life in college too.

My mind raced toward annoyance, but something stopped me. A song I'd never heard before caught my attention. It started slowly and built momentum. I closed my eyes and swayed my hips, suddenly thankful that Sophie had brought me here. She had introduced me to many new people and places over the years and she had never abandoned me. She was close by and simply enjoying a dance with her new boyfriend.

The song was about Boston, but the words hardly mattered. The offbeat synchronization ebbed and flowed from gentle to intense, and back to gentle. I rarely liked unfamiliar songs, but I loved this one.

I kept my eyes closed and tuned inwards. It was late Saturday night and I was awake. More than awake, I was standing. More than standing, I was dancing. The absence of narcolepsy was a powerful physical sensation.

My mind sent the commands to my arms and legs. My hips floated effortlessly and my knees bent and straightened perfectly. My head sat comfortably on my neck. No whiplash; no fog. It was all woven together neatly – a perfect pattern of existence.

A few images flashed in my mind – the stern face of one of my law professors, my limbs crumbled with cataplexy, the orange pill bottles on my bedside stand, Taylor looking at me like a street beggar. These negative images moved quickly, as though on their way out. At least for now, none of that mattered.

Pure uninhibited grace washed over me like a waterfall, taking with it the pent-up anger, sadness and frustration.

I'd managed to entirely tune out sensations of annoyance about Sophie and Todd's public displays of affection and in doing so, discovered a very peaceful place. Perhaps this space had always been there, but I'd never been before. I'd never been in awe of standing. I'd never closed my eyes and thought, *this* is special and worth celebrating. This was a form of freedom, only experienced from the knowledge of what it was like to have these things taken away.

When the song ended, I opened my eyes a changed person. Sophie smiled at me and I smiled back, from a new place. Leaving the dark underground club later that night, I beamed ear to ear.

"I had the best time," I told Sophie and Todd, meaning it like never before.

"I'm so glad," Sophie said.

I didn't try to explain what had happened to me. They were still drunk, I was still sober, and I didn't know exactly what this epiphany meant. It was nothing I'd ever felt before. It was a whole new way of thinking. I could direct my mind away from annoyance to happiness. It seemed transferable. If I could access this space in a sticky hot basement bar, maybe I could find it anywhere. I'd always thought my emotions were uncontrollable. That night, I'd somehow steered myself to joy.

One of the first days back to school in the new year, I stumbled into my bedroom totally exhausted after a long day of classes and fell asleep face down and butt up.

I never sleep on my stomach, I thought right before my ability to think suctioned into darkness. It was only supposed to be a quick nap.

When I awoke a few minutes later, a man was straddled over my body, slapping my butt. He laughed wildly, gaining momentum and pleasure with each swing.

I went to turn over to pull him off me, but I was frozen under him. I wanted to scream bloody murder and throw him across the room. My blood pumped with adrenaline, rage and disgust. I used all my might to squirm out, but nothing happened. My body was muted. Unable to move, I listened to the sound, like ferocious clapping at a sports game. I felt the numbing sting of this unknown hand slapping me. The context was nauseating – his hand and my butt. His rhythm beat down on my heart, speeding its pace to an unnaturally fast pace for a waking heart.

The discomfort was unbearable. Unable to move physically, my mind somehow departed my body and hovered above the scene with a bird's-eye view.

From there, I saw my attacker, his body disproportionally long and lean, like an El Greco figure. He wore a black and white leotard – a bizarre court jester costume. I recognized his face.

John? A classmate from law school that I believed had a crush on me. How had he gotten into my apartment and what the hell was he wearing? He'd always seemed like a nice harmless guy.

I shuddered in disgust and wished I could dive head first off the side of my bed into an abyss. I didn't care where the abyss took me. I didn't care if my skull hit the hardwood floor or I fell into nothingness and never re-turned. I just needed out. I'd rather not exist at all than be trapped under this hyena taking sexual pleasure in slapping my butt.

I imagined going over the edge of my bed, head first, the cool air spread-ing over my cheeks and whipping through my hair. I was surrounded by nothing, and unsure of where I was going, free falling, totally out of control, but most importantly, out of *his* control.'

I don't know when he left, but when my mind surfaced, I was face down on my bed and he was gone. I climbed off my bed right away, still thinking I had to get away. Nausea overwhelmed me. I stumbled to the bathroom and sank down in front of the toilet, hoping to purge him from me.

I gasped for air and placed my fingers down my throat, dry heaving and spitting up saliva into the toilet. I tried again, but my hand began shaking in my mouth. I crumpled down to sit eye level with the toilet bowl and leaned back against the cool bathroom tiles, my body was hot and throbbing fast. I could still hear the echoes of the slaps. His presence was still inside me when I realized what had happened.

I looked aimlessly around the black and white tiled bathroom, as the mental puzzle pieces came together slowly.

I wouldn't need to check the locks or windows of my apartment. He hadn't broken in. I wouldn't need to tell the police or tell anyone for that matter. He hadn't done anything wrong. In fact, *he* had never been there. I realized that he had been a figment of my imagination, come to terrorize my nap. He was a hallucination of narcolepsy.

My eyes closed and tears streamed uncontrollably down my cheeks. Eventually, I picked myself off the floor and walked feebly back to my bedroom. Seeing my bed, I turned around and walked to the living room. I couldn't face that space right away. What if he came back?

Tracy was studying at the dining room table. It was just past 6 p.m.

"What's up chica?"

I sat down across from her, hunched over slightly. "I, ah, had a bad nightmare."

"Aw, I'm sorry." She returned to typing. "You look like you saw a ghost."

"It was bad."

What else could I say? The slapping was shameful; I didn't want to tell her about that. Plus, I didn't think she'd get it if I tried to explain and then, I'd be frustrated on another level and that was the last thing I needed. Better to leave it unsaid. Her presence was comforting, as we sat in silence and I re-calibrated to this reality.

Later that spring, a friend invited me to a concert at the Toad, another small dark bar in Cambridge. The band was good, but not really my style. I was hanging out with a different circle of friends. They weren't very welcoming, but I hardly cared. I was happy to be out. I ordered Diet Coke and swayed in my seat with pleasure. I accessed the same place in my mind where I'd found joy at the concert with Sophie.

This was freedom from the bad times, and so I stayed out later than I should have. Arriving home past 1 a.m., I realized I didn't have time for two doses of medication.

I had to be up early the next morning as I was one of the coordinators of the Intellectual Property Symposium at school that day. I had to pack to go away for a weekend with Dad and Diana. Dad had signed the three of us up for a Narcolepsy Network conference in Albany, New York. I was nervous about the conference but excited to see Dad and Diana. Dad's doctor had adjusted his medications and stabilized his heart without a transplant, so everyone was in good spirits.

I packed my bag as quickly as possible, but ended up only taking one dose of Xyrem. In the morning, I awoke with more ease than if I'd gotten both doses. No nausea or dizziness. I rushed to put on my new black suit for the symposium. Having lost 30 pounds from August to December of 2007, I owned business suits ranging from size 12 to 6, but even the size 6 had become ridiculously baggy, so I had recently purchased a size 4 suit on clearance at the Loft. It wasn't the greatest fit, but the price was right.

I met my student volunteers at the Intellectual Property club office at school and we scurried to get the tables set up before the guests arrived.

The day flew by, I socialized and drank lots of coffee. Tiredness crept in early but I stayed active by moving around to get through the day.

Dad and Diana arrived on campus at 3:30 p.m., at the closing of the symposium. I slept most of the drive to Albany. Arriving at the Marriot, I began second guessing this trip. The hotel was nice but when I saw the narcolepsy conference registration desk in the lobby, I panicked. I didn't want to meet the people at the desk. Luckily, Dad and Diana didn't notice the conference check-in table, so we proceeded to the elevators and our hotel rooms without meeting any other people with narcolepsy on our way.

Dad knew of a great Italian restaurant in Albany. It was only five blocks away and we all loved Italian food. We walked there and sat at a white linen covered table. I enjoyed every bite of my eggplant parmesan.

While considering dessert options, my head began to tingle. The restaurant had gotten very warm and I sensed that cataplexy was close. When we were getting ready to leave, I knew I needed to explain what was going on, if there was any chance I'd make it back to the hotel without falling.

"I think I may have a cataplexy attack. When we leave, I'll walk ahead. Don't engage me. Just walk behind me."

I could tell they were confused. "Should we call a cab?" Dad asked.

"It's five blocks," I snapped.

"I know, but…"

"It's okay Dad. Just stay behind me. No talking."

Maybe I should have agreed to the ride, but interacting with the taxi driver would have likely triggered my cataplexy too.

I stood up first, resting my hands on the table for support. My vision blurred and my sense of space wobbled. What if the waiter or hostess spoke to me? I feared that any social interaction might cause my cataplexy. I took a deep breath, turned and started walking.

I rushed past the hostess and out the front door with my eyes turned down to avoid eye contact. Dad and Diana followed in silence. I walked slowly along the concrete sidewalk toward the hotel, the weakness was strong and close, waiting to push the "release" button and drop me.

I kept my head down, walking through the hotel lobby and into the elevator. On the ride to the 10th floor, we were silent. I watched the floor numbers rise. When the elevator stopped, I exited first and focused my gaze on the crimson red carpet. When I turned the corner onto the final stretch to our rooms, I reached into my purse for my key card, thinking: *I'm almost there! I made it!*

The small satisfaction flipped the switch. I collapsed with my torso over my legs. My key card fell from my hand onto the carpet.

"Tom, what do we do?" Diana's voice was close. She must have knelt next to me. She didn't touch me. I tried moving, but couldn't lift a finger or toe.

"I don't know. Julie?" Dad's voice was close, too.

I wasn't sure I was okay, but I wanted to tell them I was "there." I couldn't breathe well in this hunched position. I tried inhaling deeper but even this was out of my control.

Could I suffocate?

Experiencing life through a pinhole of consciousness alone, without any physicality to back it up, I was so far from myself and wondered which shore I was closer to – life or death?

I was fighting to move with all my might, when a door handle clicked. Someone in a nearby room must've heard Dad and Diana's panicked voices. I didn't want a stranger to see me. They'd be alarmed. Luckily, as the door hinge squeaked open, my strength re-surged through my fingers and toes, and back into my body. I gasped for air and blinked my eyes open. In the corner of my eye, I saw a woman looking down at me. I grabbed my key card, and jetted to my room, not saying a word to anyone.

I unlocked my door furiously, and walked directly to my bed. Dad and

Diana caught the open door behind me and followed.

"Julie, are you okay?" Diana asked. "Was that the cata…"

"Yeah, just leave me alone," I slurred in a haze of exhaustion.

"Are you sure?"

"Yes. Leave!"

"Call us if you need anything."

My consciousness fizzled out before the door shut behind them. I awoke about 30 minutes later from a fitful, thrashing, dream-filled sleep. Past 11 p.m., it was time to go to bed to get up for the conference in the morning.

I changed into my pajamas and mixed my Xyrem, thinking about the hallway fall. I shouldn't have snapped at Diana. Hopefully I wouldn't cross paths with the woman who'd opened her neighboring door. I wanted to bury the incident and never think or talk of it again.

I reflected on the past 24 hours. I'd gone to the concert at the Toad and had such an amazing time, but didn't get both doses of my Xyrem, which made the next day a struggle and ultimately, led me to kiss the hotel carpet. I was determined to live my life to its fullest, but didn't want to be reckless. It was a fine line. I realized that, more than ever, my choices had very real consequences.

The next morning, I was hesitant to go to breakfast. I'd yet to meet anyone related to the conference. Dad and Diana were in good spirits on the way downstairs and thankfully no one mentioned the incident from the night before.

We sat at a breakfast table with a husband and wife in their late 30s. I kept quiet, eating a light breakfast of fruit; I rarely ate in the morning anymore between feeling nauseated from my Xyrem and without appetite from my Provigil. Diana launched into conversation with our tablemates, asking them where they were from and discussing the hotel, the weather, our drives to the conference.

"Well, I don't drive," the woman said. "So he does all the driving now, since I was diagnosed with narcolepsy."

She was the one with narcolepsy – interesting. They both appeared normal, like us. The conversation stalled. Was it my turn to reveal myself? The silence was uncomfortable. I didn't want to talk about me. I sighed heavily and looked away. Diana and Dad kept quiet.

"I have narcolepsy too," I said under my breath. Now it was out there.

"Oh, do you drive?" the woman asked.

I nodded. The question had never occurred to me. Why wouldn't I drive? How could I not drive? I had to get to school everyday.

We exchanged a bit more about our experiences. Hers had developed quickly, after suffering a head injury in a car accident. I explained that I wasn't sure what caused mine, but that it had developed slowly compared to hers.

As the day continued, I became more comfortable saying I had narcolepsy. It wasn't the end of the conversation here, just the beginning. I learned that some people didn't like the term narcoleptic, and preferred the acronym PWN, short for person with narcolepsy.

People continued to ask me if I drove, which struck me as strange. No one had ever questioned my ability to drive before and I couldn't imagine losing my freedom to hop in my car and take myself where I needed to go. I got used to telling people that I was on Xyrem, which was normal here; a life improving medication, not the date rape drug.

Saturday afternoon, while walking through the lobby, I saw an older man sitting on the floor, slouched against the wall, eyes fluttering. He must have had a cataplexy attack. A woman sat at his side supporting his head, possibly his wife. I looked away quickly. I'd collapsed across the same crimson carpet upstairs the night before. Thankfully, my fall was more discreet.

During a conference session, an older woman in her 70s tried to ask a question. With eyes shut, neck shaking, jaw slackening, and slurred words, it was obvious she was struggling hard against cataplexy. It was painful to watch and I turned away.

I didn't want to be subjected to watching her body fall apart. Part of my aversion was knowing what it was like myself, on the inside, and not wanting to watch someone else suffer. But I also felt repulsion. I wanted to tell her to hide herself. It was too much for me. I hated to identify with this.

On Sunday morning, Dad came into my hotel room to talk over the logistics of the conference and the drive home. He turned to leave, then stopped at the door and walked back toward me. Had he forgotten something?

"I'm so proud of you, Jules." He opened his arms to hug me, which was strange. He wasn't much of a hugger. He had always been sort of an awkward dad – not the touchy-feely type.

He hugged me tightly and then his body began to shake and I realized he was crying. Weeping, really. He convulsed in my arms. I'd never seen him cry – never mind felt him cry. It made me so sad, I didn't want to hug anymore.

"I'm so sorry. I'm so sorry," he repeated between sobs.

"It's okay, Dad."

He finally let me go and sat on the edge of my bed, rocking back and forth and clasping his hands tightly.

It was a place he'd seen me many times. He'd listened patiently to my hopeless sobs, most recently with the breakup. I sat next to him on the bed, unsure of what to say or do.

"I didn't understand before, but I get it now," he finally said, "It's much worse than I realized."

Funny, I thought he'd understood my narcolepsy better than anyone else, but now he thought he got it.

"It's not your fault," I said.

"But it's not fair. You're so young."

"It's going to be okay, Daddy." This was a white lie and we both knew it, but what else could I say?

Eventually, he calmed down and left. I looked around the bare hotel room and finished folding my clothes into my suitcase in silence.

The conference had a big effect on Dad, perhaps bigger than it had had on me. Now, he had his own burden – to love someone deeply, his youngest child, his Fabulous Jules, and watch her navigate a serious illness. He'd always been my knight in shining armor, helping me through all my lowest points, but he couldn't save me from narcolepsy.

N ot a day went by that I didn't think about exercising. It had been a part of my daily routine and self esteem since age five, my escape route from my troubles. Now, I needed an outlet more than ever, but the thought of going to the gym made me anxious. I didn't have the energy to trample on the treadmill like before. I still wanted to do something, like yoga or Pilates, but walking past the treadmills to get to the yoga studio at my gym was like walking past my prior life – the stronger, healthier version of my past.

I was thinner now, unhealthily skinny. Peach fuzz grew on my cheeks, something Mom had warned me when I was younger was as sign of anorexia. I wasn't anorexic but I wasn't healthy.

I looked into joining a yoga studio that wouldn't have treadmills lined up outside the classroom. I arrived at one to find out they only offered "hot yoga." I left quickly. I didn't need heat to make my heart race, I had daytime stimulants for that.

"Best of Boston" listed a fancy gym as having the best yoga, so I decided to check it out.

"Don't you want to see the weights and cardio?" my tour guide asked.

"No thanks. You've seen one treadmill, you've seen them all." I kept walking, past the exercise room glass doors.

"But there's a beautiful view of the Boston Common."

"I'm sure. Can I see the squash courts?"

My tour guide was confused. I'm sure most people joined for the equipment. Not me. I was thrilled to learn that the yoga studio was on its own floor, separate from the rest of the gym, so I could go in and out without passing a treadmill. I joined immediately.

Soon after that, one of my best friends from college, Mia, visited from San Francisco during my law school spring break. Her big blue eyes and long blond hair glistened like a ray of Californian sunshine on my life. We spent the week together exploring museums, trying new restaurants, and attending yoga classes, like Yin Yoga.

The yoga studio smelled of warm wood and lavender.

"You've set this time aside to be here, so really be here." The teacher's voice was soothing.

Mia and I decided to try Yin Yoga because the description sounded easier than the active flow yoga classes. In Yin Yoga, we held stretching positions for three to four minutes on each side.

"Now place your right shin parallel to the top of the mat."

We contorted our bodies into "pigeon pose." This same stretch had been a big part of my physical therapy regimen last summer.

Within 10 seconds, a wave of nausea came over me. I'd always hated pigeon pose. Holding it for 30 seconds was hard enough. *There is NO way I will be able to hold this for four minutes*, I thought. I squirmed, hoping to find relief.

"Notice the sensations that arise in this pose," the calm instructor said.

My sensations were screaming at me like an urgent alarm. *Reject! Reject!*

"As long as you aren't experiencing sharp pain, you are okay. Dull aching pain is healthy. We're working into the connective tissues."

My pain wasn't sharp, but the dull aching was unbearable.

"All sensations are shifting. Stay in the moment with the discomfort. Notice it shift. Pay attention."

Yeah right, I thought. *This lady is nuts.*

Unable to think about anything else, I paid attention to my escalating discomfort. I opened my mouth and let out an exasperated sigh, a dragon's flames of discomfort in my breath.

"This position can bring anger to the surface. Pay attention to that, too."

No kidding.

Then, after about three minutes of pure hell, the raging calmed. I still laid in pigeon pose, but the alarms stopped sounding quite so loudly. The tension released a bit. Not entirely, but enough so that I could comfortably stay for another minute.

As the class progressed, each pose seemed harder that the one before. It was an hour and half of torture.

"I love it!" Mia exclaimed after class.

"Yeah, me too." I said, surprising myself.

Truthfully, I loved parts of it – the teacher, the scent of the room, the relaxing music. It certainly wasn't easy, but it made a deep impression upon me and how I experienced my body.

Mia and I returned two days later for our second Yin Yoga class. It was just as disquieting as the first. Folding over my right shin into pigeon pose, I reminded myself that the sensation would shift. "It will pass, it will pass," I repeated. I held on to this solace tightly to get through the unfathomable discomfort.

The teacher said our minds could be in motion even though our bodies remained in one position, which made me think about how I'd been trapped by the physical sensations of nausea, headaches and cataplexy. Perhaps if I paid attention to those moments of discomfort, I could see if they shifted too. My discomfort would pass, and knowing this, made it easier to get through.

There was something freeing about the Yin Yoga philosophy of staying in the moment. It reminded me of the space I'd tapped into while dancing with Sophie. After class, Mia and I discussed how this had affected both of us. We loved talking about various aspects of life philosophy. We connected on so many levels with ease.

Over dinner one night, we finally delved into the nitty-gritty details of my new life with narcolepsy, including the medication scheduling and the side effects.

"Well aren't there other options?" Mia asked.

I quickly became overwhelmed trying to explain. I didn't want to be a Debbie Downer, but she was looking for quick fixes. I knew she wanted nothing more than to help, yet I felt slightly insulted by her simplistic suggestions to improve things, as if I hadn't thought of those ideas.

Mia always looked for the positive, which is why I loved her so much. In college, she brought me up when I was down. Now, I discarded all of her suggestions, saying, "I'm sorry, but it's not that easy."

She was also a very patient listener. After a few hours of conversation, I'd finally painted a more accurate picture of my reality for her. Neurological illness was outside both of our realm of understanding. We were art history lovers, not exactly scientists or medical experts.

Over dessert, she became quiet. I looked up from my plate to see her staring off into space, her blue eyes glazed over with emotion. Teardrops fell delicately down her porcelain cheeks. I hadn't meant to upset her, but it was the first time I knew she understood a piece of my pain. Seeing her hold my pain hurt too, like seeing Dad cry. I didn't want to upset my loved ones, but I couldn't carry this alone.

FIFTEEN
GHOSTS

WHEN PEOPLE HAVE SOMETHING shameful to hide, they get good at finding hiding spots. I was no exception. Hiding my daytime naps became a priority every day. A private room with a locked door was ideal, which is why I studied in the Intellectual Property group's office so often. The office was two adjoining rooms, one with a conference table, the other with a big desk and refrigerator. Six group leaders had keys to the office but I was the only one who used it regularly.

One early evening, while studying for my spring finals, my Constitutional Law II textbook, notes, outlines, flashcards and computer were spread across the conference table. Con Law II was my favorite class, revealing the political side of Supreme Court decisions, but inevitably, I put my head down and fell asleep.

A few minutes later, I awoke to keys jingling outside the office. Maybe one of the other group leaders was coming to get a book or use the mini fridge.

Good timing, I thought as I was just waking up. All I had to do was sit up and appear normal.

I tried to sit up but my left cheek lay cemented against my arms over the table. The door was on my right, so in order to see who was coming in, I needed to lift my head long enough to at least turn over onto my right cheek. I tried lifting again. I pulled with neck muscles pulsing. It was no use. A gargantuan force held me down.

The doorknob rattled. Perhaps it was the cleaning staff coming to take out the trash. I pushed with all my might. Being caught waking up would be unbearably embarrassing.

During the struggle, a strong electric vibration surged up my back. My neck muscles shook violently, totally outside of human experience. Maybe my hand or foot *was* caught in an electrical outlet. The shock moved through me for a few seconds, maybe longer, I wasn't sure – I was only conscious for a snapshot of extreme discomfort, before my mind washed back into darkness.

The keys jingled again. With all my might, I lifted my head off of my hand-pillow and squinted at the door.

Thump.

My head dropped against the table. I tried to look at the door again – I *needed* to see who was coming.

Then, everything was silent. No keys, no doorknob, no resistance, no cement, no electric shock. New and different sensations flooded my body: raging, racing, boiling, gasping, surging. My body lit with adrenaline pumping through my veins. My head lifted and dipped like a buoy in choppy water, as my muscles came and went.

I breathed deeply after the prolonged inability to do so. My eyes darted to the door handle. Had someone been outside? My memory of the sound was fresh and real, but no one had come in. Maybe I'd heard keys jingling outside a neighboring office door and got confused. My spine was numb from the odd electric pulsation. My thought process was slow and eventually I realized that this was probably just another imaginary intruder.

The Intellectual Property group's office, once locked, was an incredible hiding place during my second and third years at law school, though even there, the visitors found me. Sleep invaded my day, as an unwelcoming guest – terrorizing and soul-sucking. The Xyrem substantially reduced the number of visitors in the night, but daytime naps were still fair game for sleep paralysis and hypnagogic hallucinations.

I looked at my books and notes – the pile of inanimate words that needed to enter my brain for my exam the next day. My head was like a stormy wasteland between dreams and nightmares. How was it that the *fake* world seemed so much more real to me than reality?

I was not sure how to proceed, to move from the surreal to the real. It was a war between my own body and mind playing tricks on me. I wanted to move on and re-concentrate on Constitutional Law, but a crucial piece of me was gone.

I was both the predator and victim of the intrusion. I should've been able to move back into reality seamlessly. My exam was the next day and I was far from prepared. My insatiable hunger to succeed that had pushed me through long arduous study sessions in high school and college felt like a past lifetime. I had all the same pressures now, but I might as well have been dead. I decided to go home and call it a night. I'd get up very early to try to cram in as much studying as possible before the exam.

It was still dark out when my alarm went off the next morning. I'd barely studied and my mind raced forward to the tasks ahead. I lifted my arm. It was weak as if someone had carved the flesh off of my bones in the night. Then, I noticed dampness on my bed. Was this wetness from me? I touched my lips.

I didn't know if it was saliva or vomit, but it grossed me out. I burped over and over, while climbing off my bed and looking back at the circle of wetness below my pillow.

A few snapshot images came back to me. I'd woken up in the middle of the night to take my second dose of medication and was hungry. Since I couldn't eat two hours before going to bed, sometimes I got hungry during the night. Last night, I went to the kitchen for Cheez-It crackers. I knew this was against the rules, but the compulsion to eat was overpowering. I was still drugged from my first dose of Xyrem.

After finishing the Cheez-Its, I took my second dose of medication even though I'd just eaten. There was no time to spare because I had to get up early to study for my exam. Cheez-Its and medication were not a good combination. I tossed feverishly around until I was finally swept back into my blacked out, sedated sleep.

I knew better than to eat on my medication. Yet somehow the strict rules had lost their pull over me. My power was drained by the struggle between my sickness and my life.

I dressed slowly. I wanted to crumble back into bed, but looking at it reminded me that I couldn't – it was wet and shameful. I had to step forward, my mind stuck in my sickness, body heading on to exam. "Just keep going," I told myself.

I've heard that sometimes a version of you must die before another more enlightened version can be born. I think that's true after watching the corpse of myself walk around law school during my second and third years of law school.

It's easy to see why I was so unaware of my extremely poor state of health for so long. It was almost undetectable from the outside. As soon as I started to realize how different I was, I also began to realize that no one else could see the difference. Almost everyone saw my old self while my new self was pushed out of the picture. For a while, I liked the fact that no one could see my new self, as it was so unexpected and, frankly, *so* unwelcome.

My old self faded away slowly, yet everyone tried to keep up with her. They struggled to evoke the ghost of my old self. They spoke to someone else and loved someone else entirely. I watched in disbelief as my ghost puffed smoke and people nodded, believing the dead spirit's voice. I remember the first time I let my new self out in public.

In the spring of my second year, I scurried home one night after class to meet Mom at my apartment. It was pouring rain. I jumped in her car and we drove down the road to Harvard Medical School. Dr. Larson had invited me to present at a class with him. I could bring a guest so I invited Mom to join me.

Even in the rain, the Harvard Medical School campus was regal with matching marble buildings standing tall around a grassy quad. We found the building that matched our directions. A security guard buzzed us in. After signing in, we sat on a wooden bench and waited to be accompanied to the classroom. My heart raced and the dampness of my clothes sent a shiver down my back. Maybe this wasn't a good idea.

Mom chattered about her tennis friend's son getting married and who was invited to the wedding and who wasn't. I barely responded. The wedding gossip seemed insignificant to me.

"What's wrong, Julie?"

"I'm nervous, sorry." Mom always picked up on my mood quickly. She hadn't seen much of my cataplexy and I wasn't sure what she thought of my disorder.

Eventually Dr. Larson escorted us to the classroom and motioned for us to sit in the front row near the podium. The small, outdated stadium classroom was much less intimidating than the building's fancy exterior. About 30 adults of all ages, men and women, medical students and doctors, chatted amongst themselves before class. Announcements were made and then Dr. Larson invited me to join him at the front of the room. We sat in plastic chairs facing the audience. I placed my hands on my thighs, hoping no one would notice my slight nervous tremor. The Provigil still made me shake during big moments like this.

Dr. Larson was calm, which put me at ease. First, we discussed the progression of my early symptoms.

"I was having trouble studying," I explained, "and driving, even 15 minutes to school in the morning and – "

As I spoke, I saw an image of my car swerving out of control on the exit ramp to Dad and Diana's house in New Hampshire. I gasped. Other pictures flooded back – open car windows, the radio dial, guardrail, brakes. I blinked a few times, returning to the classroom.

"Sorry, I forgot what I was saying." I smiled to ease the awkward moment. I couldn't mention this incident. I wasn't even certain it had happened, and if it had, how had I not remembered it until now? A deep dark layer of repression and denial dropped to the floor.

Next, Dr. Larson asked, "How has narcolepsy affected your life as a busy law student?"

I paused, soaking in the broad question, then told them about the night I went to the concert at the Toad and had to be up early the next morning for the Intellectual Property symposium, and ultimately collapsed in the hotel hallway in Albany.

"I can't say I'd go back and change anything. The concert was fun, but falling was suffocating and humiliating. I guess I live in greater extremes now." Hearing myself say this was perhaps a moment of realization for me too. I looked up and saw a female student about my age, leaning forward in her seat. She appeared deep in thought. She *cared*, I could tell.

Our interview was only supposed to last 30 minutes but the students asked so many questions that it ended up being about 45 minutes before I sat back down next to Mom in the audience. Presenting for the Harvard Medical School class was more fun than I'd thought it would be. I got to talk about myself to a captive audience who listened and laughed at my jokes.

Next, Dr. Larson went through a slideshow about the neuroscience behind sleep and narcolepsy. I listened intently to his descriptions. He became very excited when he showed my sleep study results. "Julie went into REM in all five naps and spent nearly the entire time of each nap in REM sleep!"

"Hooray!" I sarcastically lifted my arms up in the air and everyone laughed. Science and reality were so different.

Next, Dr. Larson showed a video of a 9-year-old boy having cataplexy. I'd watched this video on YouTube a few times, but seeing it on the large projection screen, I cringed and closed my eyes. The boy looked so gross and unnatural as he sank and bobbed. I knew the feeling in my bones, in my muscles, and across my heart.

The discussion moved to the disease process and the current theories of why narcolepsy develops in people like myself. Any car accidents? No. Trauma to the head? Not that I could recall. Periods of heavy drug use? Definitely not. There was a moment of silence when many possibilities had been raised and discarded. Dr. Larson suggested a possible connection to upper airway infections like streptococcus or influenza, but many unanswered questions remained. This part of the presentation was depressing.

Afterwards, the students and doctors approached one by one to thank me.

"This is *so* helpful," they said. "We appreciate your willingness to share."

These were the same stories that made my friends and family look away, but here, my stories were welcome.

"Thank you for taking good care of her, doc," Mom said, shaking Dr. Larson's hand respectfully.

"I'm sure you've heard all this plenty," he responded.

"No, not really." This was the truth. Her honesty surprised me.

I hadn't told her many of these stories because she hadn't asked much about my narcolepsy and I hadn't pushed it upon her. I was thankful she took the time to drive down from New Hampshire to attend the class with me.

I'd described my sleep paralysis and hypnagogic hallucinations in great detail during the presentation. Mom didn't say anything about it at the time, but later that week, I received a card in the mail from her, thanking me for inviting her and stating, "I hate thinking of my baby having those terrible nightmares."

It surprised me that she'd gravitated to this part of my story. Cataplexy was much scarier, but the vivid dreams resonated strongest with her, maybe because they were more relatable.

I was still coming to terms with understanding that narcolepsy was a serious disorder myself. Not realizing that I needed, or deserved support, I hadn't asked for it from most people. Whatever small sign of support Mom offered now was welcome. She was on her own path of acceptance and understanding, which couldn't be forced along any faster than my own journey.

The Harvard Medical School presentation furthered my subconscious shifting from my old self to a new self. I'd lost my drinking lifestyle and my ability to burn the candle at both ends. I'd prided myself on having those characteristics and abilities that had been taken away from me. So what now?

During a check-in with Dean Wilson at school, we reflected back to our first meeting and how I'd so adamantly resisted her suggestion that narcolepsy may have affected my first year grades. We both laughed. I told her more about my diagnosis process and my doctor getting excited by how bad my narcolepsy was. She admitted that she was surprised to hear that my case was serious.

"I guess you just seem so put together."

I prided myself on this deception, yet it did me no favors if I wanted sympathy from people who only saw my outer skin. From Dean Wilson's perspective, and perhaps from most people's perspective, there were no signs of illness or struggle written across my forehead. I brought the act to law school, diligently planned and orchestrated the disguise, playing the part of the perfect young woman I wanted so badly to be. It never transformed me into healthy again, but it kept my dignity high, even when I was sweating, gagging, and terrorized by my hidden side of life. I wiped away the spit, sweat and tears in the bathroom. I fooled them all, but I was also fooling myself.

The MIT Faculty Club was on the top floor of a tall building in Cambridge. Expansive windows looked out onto the Charles River – providing a breathtaking view of Boston from above. Glasses of wine were served on silver trays. I asked for a Diet Coke and chatted with some younger researchers. Once a month, a group of the best Boston area neuroscientists came together to brainstorm ideas. Problems, like narcolepsy, were presented with the hope that maybe someone from outside of the immediate discipline might think of an outside-of-the-box solution. It was a think tank, a fancy brainstorming session for really smart people. Dr. Larson had asked me if I'd like to share my patient perspective and I'd eagerly accepted.

The presentation went a lot like the one at Harvard. The doctors and scientists asked lots of questions and listened intently to my responses. Afterwards, a beautiful rosemary chicken buffet dinner was served; including steaming mashed potatoes and a medley of yellow squash and red peppers. One of the younger female researchers, Laura, approached me in line and introduced herself.

"I appreciated your presentation *so* much. You probably noticed me nodding my head a lot."

I smiled politely. I hadn't noticed her, everyone had been eagerly listening.

"I understand because," she whispered, "I also have narcolepsy."

I stood frozen, holding the tongs for the chicken.

"Oh wow. Really?"

We stepped aside in the hallway, holding plates of food, chatting about our experiences. Laura was there as a researcher, finishing her Ph.D. in neurology. She also had narcolepsy with cataplexy. She was energetic, smart, well spoken, accomplished and beautiful.

After the dinner, Laura and I left the building together. It was late and I didn't know Kendall Square very well. Laura's car was parked much closer than mine, so she offered to drive me to my car and I quickly agreed. We sat in her car chatting for more than an hour. The similarities were endless: our friends' and families' reactions, our experiences with medications, and our crazy nightmares. We exchanged email addresses and promised to stay in touch. I drove home more energetic than ever.

M id-January, I squinted in the dark one night to read the time – 5 a.m. I reached for the two orange pill bottles on my side table and lifted them to make sure I'd taken both doses. One bottle was still full.

I'd set my alarm for 4 a.m., but must've slept through it. I thought through the options. If I took the second dose now, the earliest I could get up would be 9 a.m., but my first class, taught by one of my favorite professors, started at 9 a.m. I'd be *really* late. If I skipped the dose, I could get to class on time, but sleepiness and cataplexy may creep in by early afternoon or evening. I'd been on Xyrem for over a year and hated missing a dose. My tolerance for fogged mental connections was low. I had a full day of classes ahead and the thought of battling fogged mental connections was sickening. I gulped down the second dose, re-set my alarm for 9 a.m., knowing I'd be late.

I jumped out of bed at 9 a.m. and stumbled to the bathroom, still slight-ly woozy and disoriented. Arriving at school just past 9:30 a.m., the closer parking lot was full so I had to park in the far lot. Speed walking to the law school, my mind clattered with my usual inner dialogue, *You've missed half of class, Julie. What the hell is wrong with you? Get it together.*

Just outside the law school building, I closed my eyes and took a deep breath. The negative statements echoed in my mind and for once, I rec-ognized this voice for what it was – poison. I'd been scolding myself for my every misstep since being diagnosed with narcolepsy. Self-criticism had motivated me to work harder in the past, but now, I was only hurting my-self. With little-to-no positive reinforcement from others, beating myself up made no sense. If I wasn't compassionate toward myself, no one else would be either. It had to start within.

Your circumstances are unique, Julie. Just staying in school is an accomplishment, I told myself.

This voice came out of nowhere. No one had suggested this, but I had a growing suspicion that outside of this bubble, and in the long run, staying in school with narcolepsy was a success. I wasn't sure I believed this fully, but I had to try. I vowed to muffle the negative self-talk and joined class 40 minutes late, knowing I was doing my best.

That spring, I pushed open the workout room doors at my gym and climbed onto a stationary bike. I began pedaling and reading a book when I noticed a treadmill open up in the corner, next to two panels of glass windows overlooking the Boston Common. I quickly gravitated to the treadmill and walked slowly while reading. I was so enthralled with my book that time passed quickly. Before I knew it, the treadmill turned off automatically after an hour.

I restarted it and glanced out onto the Boston Common. The sun was dipping behind the skyscrapers to my left. The night rose in navy blue on my right. I put down my book to soak in the view. All at once, the street lamps of the Boston Common lit up by the hundreds – through the various footpaths. It looked like sheets of stars covering the floor while above, the real stars were just coming out too. The whole world around me seemed to sparkle – stars on the ceiling and floor of the universe.

I turned up the speed to a light jog. Beads of sweat formed on my forehead. It had been a long time since I'd felt sweat clinging to me from a work out.

After 10 minutes of jogging, I reduced the speed to zero and stepped off the treadmill, smiling. Ten minutes wasn't much, but it was everything to me on that day. I didn't have the energy or desire to trample along like I used to for three to seven miles. I didn't need to go longer or harder. Ten minutes was perfect.

In April, Sophie hosted her birthday party at a fun Ethiopian restaurant with a large group of girlfriends – about 20 of us total. I'd just met up with Laura that afternoon and was running a few minutes late.

When I arrived, I leaned in for a big hug. "Happy Birthday! Sorry I'm late, I met up with that narcolepsy lady earlier."

Sophie hugged me. "Thanks. How did it go?"

"Great! Time flew. I just left her to come here, after three hours in Starbucks."

"You seem radiant." Sophie was genuinely excited for me to make friends with an inspiring woman with narcolepsy.

"Red or white?" one of Sophie's high school friends held up a bottle of wine.

"Oh, no thank you," I replied. Next time I saw the waitress, I ordered a Diet Coke. I was parched.

When the waitress returned to take dinner orders, without my Diet Coke, I ordered and added, "And can I please get that Diet Coke?"

Our entrees arrived 20 minutes later, but there was still no Diet Coke. I watched our waitress closely, as she chatted with a co-worker across the room. The bottles of wine had come quickly but my soda was overlooked, which annoyed me. My head began to tingle – the first sign of cataplexy. I leaned back in my chair in case of weakness. After a few moments, the fuzziness passed.

"Sophie, could you ask the waitress for my Diet Coke? I've asked twice, and I'm afraid walking over to ask again might cause cataplexy."

"Of course." Sophie went to the waitress, on a mission to get my drink. Within minutes, my Diet Coke arrived. *Finally.* As the evening progressed, a dissonance between myself and the rest of the table grew more obvious. The wine relaxed them into a different world. No one paid attention to the time or the check that arrived. The clicking clock brought on increasing fogginess. I masked my fatigue as well as I could behind a silent smile.

Leaving the restaurant, Sophie mentioned going out dancing. I was exhausted but I couldn't abandon her on her birthday. She was my rock, not to mention my side-kick for all my birthday adventures in years past. I went along to the nearby dance club.

Schoolwork was piling up and my sleepiness was terrible, but I rose to the occasion, reaching a point of over-exhaustion that closely bordered on delirium. In some strange alternate reality, I had a good time. I loved dancing and I loved Sophie. She was one of the best friends I'd ever had, supporting and accepting me during my lowest points with narcolepsy. We danced until 1 a.m. Even though I was sober, I knew I would pay for this the next day. I was exerting energy I didn't have, taking out a loan on life that I couldn't repay.

SIXTEEN
JUST A DREAM

A FEW DAYS LATER, Dad called to talk about the bar exam preparation class. The registration deadline was quickly approaching.

"Not one bone in my body wants to take the bar exam," I told him, and not for the first time.

"I know, but you just have to get through this one final step."

The past three years had been a dark time, and I was more than ready for the light at the end of the tunnel. Only problem was, I was having a hard time finding the light.

"Then what? Become a lawyer?" Not one bone in my body wanted that either.

The last time Dad and I talked about my career future, I was in college and he'd convinced me to go to law school to study art law. I'd loved art law and also became passionate about health law after my diagnosis. However, I wasn't sure I wanted to be a lawyer now. After my unsuccessful second year interview season, I hadn't pursued many other career options. I'd been focusing on getting through one day at a time, which had kept me quite busy between narcolepsy and law school.

Regardless, in just a couple of months, at age 25, I would walk in a cap and gown to receive my Juris Doctor degree from Boston College Law School. And after that, I had no clue.

The bar exam loomed like a fate worse than death, but it was my only option. Everyone takes the bar at the end of law school. I'd be foolish not to get it over with now, while everything was "fresh" in my head, while all my friends were taking it. Yet my indifference to my legal career was approaching repulsion. Even graduating was tainted by the bar exam. My friend Mia wanted to come from California to celebrate my graduation. Celebrate? What was there to celebrate? I would be free for one weekend, then return to school for the grand finale. Knowing the bar was around the corner, I didn't feel like celebrating.

"Dad, I don't know if I can keep doing this."

He was confused. Until today, I guess I hadn't said it so directly, although it had been growing in my heart for a while, like a barnacle, uninvited and consistent. On many occasions, I'd told him I was dreading the bar and that I was not happy whatsoever. Neither of us had gone so far as to suggest any alternative. I'd hoped he would sense the negativity in my voice, the premeditated resentment storming and suggest, "How about you not take the bar?"

I would fight the suggestion at first and then eventually give in. But he never brought it up, so neither did I, until now.

"I'm sorry, Julie, you're going to have to get a job eventually."

He was exasperated, which was very unlike him, and why was he apologizing? I was the one who was sorry for my wandering mind and numbed passion for the law firm career we'd dreamed up together, the perfect tribute of following in his footsteps.

"I know I have to get a job, I just don't want a law job."

"Why not a law job?"

I believed I could be a lawyer, so long as I would be willing to sacrifice everything for it, my health, sanity, friendships, everything. I didn't want it that badly. What had changed? For one thing, time. My medications had improved my wakefulness, giving me between four to six productive hours at a time, in which I could tackle the world. I had to prioritize this time carefully, doing the most important things first.

Fogginess was inevitable each day. Usually in the late afternoon or early evening it rolled in, demanding sleep. If I was in a place conducive to napping, the fogginess could resolve itself quickly within 15 to 45 minutes. Some naps were rejuvenating. Others were terrorizing with hypnagogic hallucinations and sleep paralysis that left me mentally drained.

If I couldn't nap, I was able to perform less demanding functions, like eating, socializing, walking around, and checking my email. I let calls go to voicemail and put off anything requiring effort for "later."

After the first energy dip, I'd often have an hour or two of wakefulness before the tide rolled in again. Inevitably, most days ended in a washout of half-written emails, unreturned phone calls and untouched homework assignments. I had good intentions but terrible follow through.

I'd managed to get through law school in pockets of wakefulness, but something else significant had changed – something I didn't realize until Dad's next comment.

"A job may not always be fulfilling, Julie, sometimes it's just a way to get by."

I knew many people who didn't care for their jobs. Every job I'd ever had was like this. These jobs facilitated other areas of fulfillment and interest. I understood this pattern perfectly and always accepted it for myself too.

Yet, Dad's voice echoed times past. The pep talks lined up quickly in my memory and I heard all of them at once now. "Just get through this one last year," "Keep moving forward," "Only one more month," "One more week," "You'll just have to keep going."

Usually this advice motivated me to get over the next big hump, but today, for the first time, I was weary of his survival tactics. I'd been going like this, just "getting through," my entire life. I closed my eyes and leaned back in my chair, bewildered and lost.

A vivid image flashed in my mind of a pale feeble female body propped up in a hospital bed, her eyes glassed over like white marbles. I had no idea where this image came from, but I was sure that the woman was in the hospital because she had become so numb to life and eventually looked to end her existence. Even though her body barely remained alive, her marble eyes revealed to me that her soul was dead and gone.

I'd never seen anything so powerful and scary in my mind's eye while awake.

I opened my eyes to get away from the nightmarish vision, and was back in the present, gripping my cell phone tight to my ear.

"You there?" I said softly.

"Mhm," he sounded slightly upset.

"I don't know how to explain this exactly," I paused, "but if I keep going like this, there will come a day when you'll be happy I'm alive at all."

I'd never felt in danger of killing myself, nor threatened to do so, yet the vision was an omen. This was me in the future if I kept going doing down this path of fulfilling the expectations and dreams of others detached from my reality of narcolepsy and life interests and passions. I had to stand up for myself and find a life worth living. I had to depart. It was a choice between life and death.

I'd already let pieces of my soul go and needed to re-find them. Narcolepsy kept me from working longer hours than others, but it hadn't interfered with my ability to be passionate and work hard in my pockets of good time, and knowing that passion plus hard work was me at my best, I believed it was possible for me to be successful in some sense of the word.

"What do you plan on doing, Julie?"

Good question. A prolonged silence buzzed between us while I searched for an answer.

I pushed my cell phone close against my ear, getting as close as possible to Dad. He was so patient and usually understood me better than anyone. Today, we were a million miles apart.

Eventually, I spoke. "Dad, can we talk about this later?"

"Okay, Jules. Love you."

"Love you, too."

I shifted in my desk chair for a few minutes before deciding to drive home. Ten minutes later, I redialed him while driving on the highway.

"Dad, I want to write."

"Write what?"

"Maybe a book, like my health law professor suggested."

I'd told him about this idea before. My health law professor had encouraged me to turn a paper I'd written about rare disease drug policy into a book. She said it was the best paper she'd ever received in all her time at BC Law and Harvard Law. Dad had been proud of my accomplishment but when I'd brought up her idea of turning the paper into a book, he'd always moved on to other topics quickly.

"Writing is just a dream, Julie, something you can pursue later in life."

My heart sank. This wasn't the response I hoped to receive. But then, I smiled. His "just a dream" word choice was ironic. Was I dreaming? If it wasn't for the fact that I was driving 70 mph down the highway, I might have second-guessed myself. Everyday, I had to sort out dreams versus reality.

Most people's dreams could be pushed aside, discarded as fantasies or put on a bucket list for later. Yet my dreams refused to wait – they were already here.

He was right, in a way, I was dreaming. My dreams had been a curse, but they'd also woken me up to my life. I couldn't just keep going like a robot. I had to find a path worth living.

I'd stopped caring about almost everyone's opinions of me by now, but still gripped tightly to Dad's approval. I desperately wanted his support, but realizing that I wasn't going to get it this time, I had to go on alone.

SEVENTEEN
RUN AWAY

A T GRADUATION, MY CLASSMATES and I lined up in alphabetical order and approached the stage to accept our diplomas. Dean Wilson was sitting on stage, but she wasn't the person handing out the diplomas. When my name was called, she rose from her seat to give me a hug. Her special congratulations caused a moment of confusion on stage since we backed up the procession line for a few seconds. Neither of us cared. On that day, I received no awards or academic honors, but the hug from Dean Wilson reminded me of how far I'd come.

Mom, Dad, Diana and Sophie all attended and after the ceremony, we took many photos. Sophie brought bubbles, so we giggled like schoolgirls blowing bubbles together to celebrate. Graduating from law school with narcolepsy was certainly not what I'd signed up for three years earlier, but I was relieved it was over. Everyone was extremely proud of me. I decided not to take the bar exam, to take on a writing career instead. Although I was still ironing out the details – no one tried stopping me. It simply wasn't discussed much in my family, which was fine by me.

Soon after graduating, my good friend from law school, Edward, said he was moving to DC and needed a roommate, so I decided to tag along. I could write anywhere and DC had always interested me.

Before securing my moving plans, I spoke with Dad. He thought it was a good idea, which surprised me, since I'd be moving far from him.

Mom was excited about the idea, especially because of all the great museums in DC. She was in the process of moving herself, from New Hampshire to Florida, so DC would be closer to her.

It was hard to tell my sister. She lived outside of Boston and although our busy schedules meant that most of our conversations were by phone, I would have been upset if *she'd* moved away. I would miss her and my two nephews so much.

"I think it's a great idea," my sister responded, "You should get away from it all."

I was shocked by her peppiness but glad she wasn't mad. What did she mean about getting away from it all?

"You've had a hard couple years with law school and narcolepsy."

Although she was right, a change of scenery wouldn't change too much. I couldn't run away from narcolepsy. I'd lived in the same apartment for four years and resided in New England my whole life. It was hard to leave, but it felt right.

Edward and I moved into a newly renovated tall marble-faced apartment building in the heart of the trendy U Street neighborhood in DC. The building had been a luxury hotel in the 1920s. Surprisingly, the rent was reasonable. Our apartment, on the third floor, was down a long hallway, far from the elevators and exits. Edward let me hang a huge Red Sox poster in the dining area and a few framed photographs I'd taken of the Boston skyline from along the Charles River.

A few weeks after settling in, soldiers arrived in my room one night and moved around me as if I wasn't there, hiding in my closet, behind my door and framed pictures on the walls. They lined the street outside my window and marched back and forth in the moonlight, maybe guarding me? Guns fired and I lay paralyzed in the crossfire, even unable to move when the soldier lifted his gun with the barrel pointing directly at me.

"Stop!" I tried to yell, but nothing came out.

Then, a loud blast exploded in my head – the loudest most painful sound I've ever heard.

A few minutes later, I opened my eyes, but was unsure of where I was. Dim views – my desk, my door, my framed law school diploma, came in and out of focus. These objects were familiar, and I knew I should know the space, but I couldn't place myself.

When I was able to move again and looked around more, it was clear that this was my bedroom, but where was that? I picked myself out of bed, walked to the door and peered into the dark hallway. There was a door to my right. I knew I should know who lived there. But who was it? I recognized the hallway but wasn't sure where it went. What building was this? What city? What state? Where were the soldiers now?

My hands roved my scalp for signs of bleeding or damage. The sensation of the blast was fresh and very real. Should I check my closet for any lingering soldiers?

Slowly everything made sense again. Edward lived behind that door. The hallway led to the living room of our apartment in Washington, DC. I lived here. My head hadn't been shot to pieces. The soldiers were just night visitors.

Edward began making many convincing appearances, too. Working from home, I often napped on the couch in the living room. One day, I heard him call my name and felt his hand on my shoulder, trying to wake me, but I couldn't move or tell him I heard him. A few minutes later, when I woke up, he was gone.

On a Sunday morning, as I was drifting in and out of sleep, a high-pitch screaming woke me with a startle – it sounded like a kid throwing a tantrum. An adult's voice echoed in, too, trying to calm the kid, I assumed. No children lived near us, but maybe one was visiting our neighbors. I went back to sleep. A few minutes later, the wailing continued. I rolled over and drifted off again.

When I woke up later, around 11 a.m., I quickly discarded the incident. As real as the screaming sounded at the time, I'd stopped trusting anything taking place around my sleep time. The kid was just another visitor.

Later, that evening, Edward asked, "Did you hear that kid screaming this morning?"

"Oh, you heard that too?" I was shocked.

"Yes, how annoying! I almost went out there to say something."

If Edward heard the kid too, then it had been real. My inability to judge dreams from reality had reached the point that I was now confusing *reality* for dreams.

That fall, I received a message from a Boston-based non-profit organization called Wake Up Narcolepsy, asking if I knew of anyone who'd like to run the Boston Marathon for narcolepsy research.

Within three minutes, I responded, "I'd like to run the marathon for narcolepsy!"

I didn't ask anyone else's opinion on the matter, or think through my own capabilities and physical restrictions. My decision to run the Boston Marathon was one of the most thoughtless decisions I've ever made.

There were some decisions I took very seriously. I weighed the pros and cons, thought through worst and best-case scenarios, belabored the main points over and over in my head and got advice from friends and family.

Then, there were times I'd made decisions without thinking. Impulse purchases and last minute, on-a-whim choices were often the decisions I regretted most, the times I'd hoped I'd kept the receipt and prayed for a forgiving return policy. Was running the marathon just a whimsical folly I'd later regret?

There were plenty of reasons why I should have said no. As a person with narcolepsy, intense exercise made me tired. Running could be dangerous with my cataplexy – as I could have muscle weakness while running and possibly fall and injure myself.

Narcolepsy had taught me to listen to my body and respect its boundaries. I was fragile, twistable, breakable and 100 percent fallible. Yet, when the opportunity came to run the Boston Marathon on behalf of people with narcolepsy, I accepted the challenge in a heartbeat.

Perhaps there are some decisions that are beyond thought, beyond logic, beyond science, and beyond health. Decisions that others can't help us make; things we must do for ourselves because if we don't, we'd only be cheating ourselves.

There would always be complications and failures. I could have sat around thinking about the "what ifs" and "maybes." Or, I could've stood up, started running and watched what happened.

I chose to run.

"You don't strike me as the marathon type," one friend responded upon hearing the news.

I opened my mouth to respond, but no words came. A bundle of nerves hit heavy at the bottom of my stomach. Until her comment, everyone had ferociously applauded my decision to train for the marathon.

"Don't you have to run another marathon to qualify first?"

Oh, it was just a misunderstanding. My friend had confused me for a "qualifier," a very different breed of human that runs marathons more seriously.

"No, no, no! I'm running for *charity*," I explained. "It's completely different. I don't have to qualify."

Attempting to paint over the awkward moment, I spoke about my training plan. It was only mid-October, so I still had six nice fat months sitting comfortably between me and my goal of 26.2 miles in April. By the end of the conversation, she agreed that this was great news.

Yet, on some level, my friend was right. I wasn't the "marathon type." Some people are born runners – it's in their DNA. I'd always been an outsider peering in on their elite runners' world.

When I ran cross-country in high school, I usually came in fifth place on our team, the last spot on varsity. Wanting to run faster and place higher, I looked to Malcolm, our school's zany art history teacher by morning, turned passionate cross-country coach by afternoon. He knew what to eat, what not to eat, what muscles to stretch, how to maximize up hills, how to avoid the impact of down hills, and how to prevent every conceivable running injury.

Malcolm was entirely invested in our success, training us to reach our individual maximum potential. One day, after a disappointing timed training run, I asked Malcolm, point blank, "What else can I do to improve?" He responded with a shrug of the shoulders. Given his extensive expertise, his muted answer spoke loudly. There was nothing else to be done. I'd reached my potential.

So what was the insurmountable gap between me and the elite pack of runners in high school? When they ran, they looked like wild gazelles lunging effortlessly, their delicate legs in a constant circular motion. It made me dizzy watching them, never mind trying to keep up with them. When I ran, my legs chafed.

Even though running did not come naturally to me, I got hooked on it as a means of getting away from my problems. The summer between my freshman and sophomore year in high school, my parents were in divorce proceedings. Running wasn't pleasant, but it was quiet. I slipped out through the cracks of anger, saying, "I'm going for a run." No one noticed. The fresh air and solitude became a therapy of sorts – precious time used to untangle what others said from how I felt.

During this first summer, I ran one and only one route. Leaving home, I traveled along the forest-lined roads toward downtown Durham, N.H. The hot summer filtered a spongy patchwork of light along the worn grey pavement road.

Downtown, at the University of New Hampshire, I jogged through packed parking lots, past dormitories and science labs, and eventually arrived at the University's track. It was wrapped around the football field, at the center of a large sports complex. I tallied my laps until I inevitably lost count, consumed by much more pressing thoughts and emotions. When fully depleted, I returned home along the same route in reverse.

The more I ran, the more I relied on this time for myself. I wasn't particularly good at relaxing. Watching TV made me anxious. Video games didn't hold my attention. Constantly in fear of "wasting my time," running forced me to get away from myself, if only for 30 minutes.

Also, the more I ran, the easier it got. Not just a little easier, *a lot* easier. My junior year in high school, I joyfully switched my fall sport from soccer to cross-country. At Brown, I'd continued running as much as possible, although during the school year, I also played women's varsity squash. Summers, I taught tennis at Harvard. No matter what sports I played, I made time for running.

For 10 years, I called myself a runner – not the gazelle-type, just the average-type – until the fall of 2007, right after my 24th birthday, when I was diagnosed with narcolepsy while also struggling with tendonitis in my knees.

While in law school, I found it difficult to work out before class or before doing my homework, since I was often less productive after hitting the gym. Now I was working as a writer at home, so I could schedule my training for the late afternoons and early evenings, after I finished my intellectual work for the day.

Before preparing for the marathon, I was in the worst shape of my life. There were no false conceptions of magically turning into a gazelle overnight.

But I had a secret weapon – an illness that had taken me to the ground and stripped me of my athleticism. I now realized this was not time wasted, but time spent building me into the person and runner I would become. Narcolepsy had become a source of inspiration – helping me to live in the moment with immediacy and gratitude. It led me to dance euphorically in the basement of a nightclub and it released me from my fears of failure. Now, it would carry me to train for a marathon. Strange as it may sound, sickness was my second chance.

When running on the treadmill before I had narcolepsy, I watched my legs and wondered whether they were chunky or normal, pale or tan, ugly or attractive. Now, I watched my legs in the full-length gym mirrors as they bent and straightened endlessly, pounding on rubber, going nowhere. I wondered why my knees held so strong sometimes and not other times. Most of all, I was in awe of them and compelled not to take my "healthier" times for granted.

I researched marathon training plans – and found a plethora of options depending on one's pace - 8 minute miles, 10 minute miles, and so on. The paces overwhelmed me. I'd run 7 minute miles in high school cross-country but that was 3.1 miles and completely different. I had no idea how fast I would be able to run 26.2 miles *with* narcolepsy.

At the bottom of one website, I found a training plan called "To Finish." I had no grand hopes or wild dreams for the marathon. My only hope was staring back at me from the computer screen, "To Finish." This was the plan for me.

EIGHTEEN
ON THIN ICE

AT THE END OF OCTOBER, it was time to start my official training. The Annual Narcolepsy Network Conference concluded on a Sunday afternoon in Jacksonville, Fla. My flight wasn't until Monday morning, so I had some time to myself.

I dressed in my workout gear and tied my old running sneakers tightly. They were dirty with remnants of red clay from the law school softball field back in Boston. There was nothing glamorous about starting training. No one cheered for me on the first day I set out toward doing something bigger than myself.

On my way out, one of the conference organizers approached me in the lobby.

"I'm about to start my marathon training!" I exclaimed with pride.

Without saying a word, she looked me up and down and leaned down to inspect my calf muscles. I giggled awkwardly, not sure what she was doing.

"Hmmm, with these legs?" she asked skeptically.

"Um, yeah?" I felt smaller and less capable then ever.

"Well, good luck!"

Maybe she was implying I might not have what it takes to run 26.2 miles. And maybe she would be right. I didn't know, but I had to try, on the only legs I had available.

I'd been in Florida all weekend, but spent the entire time indoors, cooped up in the conference rooms. Exiting the hotel was liberating.

Then a wall of heat hit me across the face. I hadn't thought about the extreme humidity in Florida. My joints began to ache. Heat and humidity really brought out my tiredness and cataplexy. I considered turning around, going upstairs and taking a nap, but I didn't want to pass by my skeptic in the hotel lobby, so I pressed on.

I walked a few minutes before picking up the pace to a lethargic jog. The Jacksonville waterfront was deserted, making it seem like a ghost town. The downtown buildings would probably be bustling during the work-week, but on a muggy Sunday afternoon, I was one of the only people outside.

There was no spunk in my step. I just moved forward either jogging or walking as time passed slowly. It was hard to breathe in the dense air.

I thought of the children and teenagers I'd met at the conference living with narcolepsy. They were some of the brightest and most mature kids I'd ever met. I was humbled and saddened when I heard their stories of how narcolepsy disrupted their young lives; falling under the spell at the young age of six or ten, diagnosed so young in life.

Many of them took medication twice a day and twice a night, like me. All this had been difficult enough to adjust to in my mid-20s – I couldn't imagine seeing my childhood through their eyes. They had their entire lives ahead of them, and there weren't any better treatments on the horizon; no miracle cure around the corner. I was determined to use my healthier times to run for them.

While on my run, I brainstormed other ways to motivate myself. I'd heard of people blogging about trips and challenges to keep friends and family updated. I'd never considered writing a blog myself. It was *so* public, but perhaps if I told the world I was running a marathon, I'd stick to it. A blog could be a good way to raise awareness about narcolepsy too.

When I returned to my hotel room, I jotted down some notes for my first post. Once home in DC, I investigated more about starting a blog. What would it be called? I emailed my friends a few choices. Julia, a friend from law school, suggested REM Runner. Perfect!

I learned that there were ways to blog anonymously, which seemed like a good option, so my full name wouldn't be connected to narcolepsy. However, remaining anonymous didn't sit right with me either.

Still unsure of the details, I went for a short run late one afternoon down 16th Street toward the White House. My marathon prep plan included walk breaks to keep my legs fresh and injury-free. The concept was new to me. Before narcolepsy, I'd viewed walking during a run as a sign of weakness. Now, I was less concerned with appearances, my goal was to finish, nothing more. I planned on training for and running the marathon by running eight minutes and walking two minutes at a time.

Around every corner in DC, I discovered interesting sculptures, foreign embassies, and lavish, gothic building facades. Boston would always be home, but I loved DC's energy. Once at the White House, I continued to the National Mall and watched the big pink sun dip down in the sky behind the Lincoln Memorial. The surrounding monuments honoring presidents and war heroes reminded me of leaders who had stood up for what they believed in. Returning home, my footsteps were light. I couldn't wait to start my blog.

Would I remain anonymous or give up my privacy? Most people thought narcolepsy was a joke about falling asleep while standing or talking. My experience had been far from this stereotype. I'd learned that many doctors were not aware of the basic symptoms. At the Narcolepsy Network conferences, I'd met individuals who went undiagnosed for 5 to 15 years, and others who had been misdiagnosed with epilepsy, depression, or schizophrenia and put on heavy medications for illnesses they didn't have. People said I was one of the "lucky ones," to be diagnosed within a few years of my symptom onset.

Once diagnosed, most PWNs, like myself, kept their condition fairly private because of the stigmas and chances of unfair discrimination.

While running, it occurred to me that we were caught in a cycle of misunderstanding, but if no one spoke up about the *real* condition, how would the cycle break?

I stopped at a busy intersection a few blocks from home to wait for a walk signal. I put my hands behind my head, gasping for air to catch my breath. I'd been sprinting without realizing it. Giving up my privacy was a big decision, but I knew, right then, I was done hiding.

The next day, I signed up to create my REM Runner blog, declaring my intentions to run the Boston Marathon while living with narcolepsy and cataplexy. I included my picture and full name, thereby placing all my cards on the table.

A month later, I was still moving slowly, making progress in a small sense by getting used to running a few times a week.

On Thanksgiving day, I was scheduled to run my first long run – seven miles. Before narcolepsy, I ran seven miles twice a week. Now, seven miles was a daunting task.

I was visiting Dad and Diana in New Hampshire for the holiday and woke up with a headache around 9 a.m. The side effects of my medications had gotten better with time, but occasionally I still woke up with a headache or nausea. I stayed in bed an extra hour and went down to the treadmill in the basement around 10 a.m.

The basement was cold and dark. Storage boxes and old furniture surrounded the treadmill. Hearing my brother's voice upstairs, I turned up the volume of my iPod to try to tune out my family momentarily and stay concentrated. My sister and nephews would arrive soon. I lost myself in the repetition and music and entered a peaceful trance state. I ran eight minutes and walked two minutes at a time.

One mile left! I told myself after an hour.

In the corner of my eye, I noticed something move. My eyes darted right, seeing my young nephew, Charlie, pop his head around the corner. With my headphones in, I hadn't heard him on the stairs.

My right foot hit the treadmill belt next, but instead of a steady strong step – my knee wobbled slightly. My chest lunged forward and my hands grabbed the handlebars instinctively. I transferred my weight into my arms and stepped off the moving belt. The surprise of seeing Charlie had caused a slight episode of cataplexy.

"Get out of here!" I yelled.

He disappeared quickly.

I shouldn't have used such a harsh tone with Charlie. He hadn't done anything wrong. I looked down at the rubber belt still spinning rapidly below. I was exhausted and this small incident brought a fear to the surface. If my body crumbled more substantially here, I could injure myself badly. I reduced the speed and walked a few minutes before finishing my last mile jogging slowly.

This was my first long run in training, and each would get longer. Sources of emotion would be inevitable – indoors and out. I wished I could turn off my feelings and stop cataplexy, but even subtle thoughts caused it at times. It was impossible not to think.

That evening, I went online and purchased a hot pink medical alert sports bracelet to wear on my training runs. I'd resisted previous suggestions that I get a medical bracelet for the past two years, believing it would brand me as sick, but experiencing cataplexy on the treadmill scared me. Although it was only a small fumble, all the bigger episodes returned quickly in my mind's eye. I would never trust my body entirely ever again.

Cataplexy while running outdoors didn't scare me as much. I could fall to the solid ground or against a tree or wall or bench. Cataplexy on the treadmill had greater consequences. I vowed to run outdoors as much as possible. DC's milder winter weather would help make this possible.

Before leaving Boston, I threw my old ratty snow boots in the dumpster behind my apartment. They wouldn't be necessary. Once relocated, I bragged to my northern friends when DC hit 75 degrees in November.

Then, in mid-December 2009, Washington DC experienced the biggest snowstorm ever to hit DC in the month of December. The "Snowpacalypse," affectively turned the city into a winter wonderland. Unprepared for a storm of this size, DC's streets went untouched for days, and sidewalks were impassable for weeks, with huge piles of snow haphazardly looming in odd places. My training had to be brought indoors.

Luckily, I traveled to Florida a few days after the Snowpacalypse, to spend the holidays with Mom. She had recently moved from New Hampshire and I was thrilled that one of my long runs coincided with this vacation.

Siesta Key Beach was three miles of evanescent white sand. Two round trips up and down the beach made a perfect 12 miles. I took off with overeager spirit in my step. Every long run from this point on would be the farthest I'd ever run. Thus, these longer distances were each minor life achievements.

The pearly white sand was interwoven with an assortment of broken shells that crunched under my sneakers. I played my iPod at half volume so I could hear the waves crashing by my side.

While weaving around various walkers, I noticed a woman in a skimpy sundress running a few feet in front of me. She ran barefoot, wearing a bathing suit under her dress. Given her lack of proper athletic gear, I didn't like that we were practically going at the same pace, so I briefly ran side by side with Beach Barbie before bumping up my speed to leave her in the dust. My competitive athletic fighting spirit was alive and well.

On my 10th mile, things got fuzzy. My knees ached and streams of salty sweat stung my eyes. I slowly became aware that people were standing at the edge of the shore, pointing and taking pictures. My eyes glazed over the tops of the waves, wondering what everyone was looking at. Then, a dolphin fin lifted out of the turquoise ocean, not 20 feet from the shore. In my last mile and a half, I saw three different dolphins gliding in the water. This should have been paradise, but instead I gasped for air and counted down high-rise hotels and lifeguard stands until reaching my final destination.

When I returned to Mom's house, my stomach was doing flips. After my shower, Mom asked if I'd like to go out for dinner.

"Yes! I just have to lie down for a second."

Truthfully, I was dizzy and something wasn't sitting right in my stomach. I curled up in bed and quickly fell into a deep void of nothingness. When my mind resurfaced, it was dark outside. I checked the clock – 8 p.m. I'd slept three hours. I stumbled out to the kitchen, rubbing my head.

"Sorry, I don't know what happened."

"It's okay, you needed your rest. Want me to fix you something?"

I nodded and grabbed two ice packs from the freezer. Mom didn't push me to talk much. I iced my swollen knees and ate dinner quietly, zoned out. Twelve miles was far – farther than I'd ever gone before, but it wasn't even half of the marathon. What had I gotten myself into?

"What if you don't finish?" Mom asked, perhaps sensing my extreme fatigue.

"Gee, thanks Mom." My eyes darted toward her with a cutting glare.

"No, that's not what I meant!" Her eyes widened like a deer in headlights. "I meant about the donation funds for research. Would the researchers still get the money?"

"I don't know."

"Julie, I didn't mean to imply – "

"Well, you did."

Perhaps it was just a mistake, but her word choice touched a sore spot. She clearly felt terrible but I didn't care to let her off the hook right away.

I took my plate to the sink and hobbled back to bed with the ice packs. The heaviness rolled over my skull quickly and I was soon out. Around midnight, I woke up, brushed my teeth, and mixed my nighttime medication doses. My frizzy hair itched against my flushed hot neck. I still didn't feel well but I needed to start my Xyrem. I'd wake up again around 4 a.m. for my second dose and again at 9 a.m. on Christmas Eve morning, having slept about 15 hours straight.

In the morning, Mom and I pretended the little scuffle never happened and moved on to celebrating Christmas. I flew home the day after.

Later, Mom wrote me a letter reiterating that she believed in me and was sure I would finish. Her support meant a lot, but ultimately, my running would have to speak for itself.

I n mid-January, I ran a 15 mile outdoor route around the National Mall in DC a few times, and up Connecticut Avenue toward the National Zoo. I'd laced my apartment key into my running shoe for the long run, but when I returned home, I forgot to put the key back on my keychain. The next day, I returned home with groceries and realized that I'd locked myself out.

Fortunately, my doorman Freddy accompanied me upstairs with the master key. To avoid silence during the elevator ride, I attempted to explain myself.

"I went for a run yesterday and – "

I sensed that Freddy wasn't listening. He probably got this a lot. As we walked down the long hallway toward my apartment, I rambled on about training to run the Boston Marathon in April.

Suddenly, Freddy lit up. "Oh, the *Boston* Marathon!"

"Well, yes, I'm from Boston so that's why I'm running that one."

"Well, I'm from Kenya, and we usually win your marathon."

I'd always noticed Freddy's cool accent but I'd never asked him where he was from.

"Not this year. Not with me in the race!"

Unlocking my door, Freddy began laughing deeply from his belly and said, "We'll see about that."

I smiled and thanked Freddy. Closing the door behind me, I could hear him chuckling down the hall.

The following week, I waltzed through the apartment building lobby carrying a big box under my arms.

"New shoes to keep up with the Kenyans!" I told Freddy.

He smiled and shook his head.

In early February, DC's second record-breaking blizzard, "Snowmageddon," left two feet of snow on the ground, with another storm threatening to come later in the week.

My running was going incredibly well. The tendonitis in my knees seemed under control and I'd even grown to almost enjoy stretching. Co-ordinating my stretching, icing, hydrating and healthy eating schedule was a challenge, but I did my best.

Managing my narcolepsy medications and symptoms at the same time added extra complication. The medications affected when I slept, ate, and drove, and each one affected my symptoms differently and had side effects – some more tolerable than others.

These drugs were not a cure for my narcolepsy, nor did they "normalize" me by any means. However they did help me to achieve a much higher quality of life. Without these treatments, my life would have been entirely under the control of cataplexy and pervasive sleepiness. This was the reality of my condition that I had never fully lived, since I was lucky enough to start treatment just as my symptoms were becoming truly disabling. Thus, I tried to balance my frustrations with these drugs with my appreciation for their existence. The drugs were a big pain, but when it came down to it – there would've been no "REM Runner" without them.

I prioritized my treatment to get the most out of my life, but the snow-storms proved problematic. I ran out of Xyrem during the snowstorm week. My next shipment was in the mail, but due to two confounding blizzards, our building didn't receive mail for a whole week.

Without Xyrem, my sleep was fragmented and restless. The first morning after not taking any, I walked into my living room and saw Edward sitting at the kitchen table. It wasn't a big deal, but I hadn't expected to see him there. This subtle surprise turned my legs to Jell-O.

Oh no. My cataplexy would only get worse throughout the day.

The options ran through my head. There was another drug I could take, an anti-depressant that would immediately wipe out my cataplexy for the day. Dr. Larson had prescribed it to use in emergencies for my cataplexy, but even a small dose of this drug left me extremely nauseated and shaky. It wasn't always worth taking it, given the side effects. I had to look at what I was supposed to do that day and decide which I preferred – extreme nausea or cataplexy.

It was a close friend's birthday and I was looking forward to celebrating with her that evening at her bar party, so I chose to take the anti-depressant over experiencing cataplexy. I sat on the couch, with strange waves of dis-quiet energy spiraling in my body. I needed to get up and go for a run, but I wasn't up to it. I wanted to be stronger than my circumstances but I was hitting a brick wall.

Of course, even if I hadn't taken this drug, I wouldn't have been able to run on the treadmill with such high chances of having cataplexy. It was a lose-lose scenario. I hoped my shipment of Xyrem would arrive soon, as DC cleaned up from the blizzards.

I'll come back stronger soon, I promised myself. I wanted this marathon badly.

The following week, I dropped off my water bottle and packet of sports energy "jelly beans" at the front desk before my 16 mile run. Freddy laughed.

"No chance. No chance." I laughed, too.

The roads were sloppy with slush leftover from last week's storms. I ran cautiously up the hills of Adams Morgan on Connecticut Avenue past the National Zoo toward the Maryland border. As planned, I ended my first seven mile loop back at my building, to hydrate and energize mid-run. I entered my building, sweating and sniffling, with flushed red cheeks. Freddy handed over my water and jellybeans.

"Now, you look like a runner. Maybe you *will* run with the Kenyans."

It was the enemy speaking the unspeakable. Smiling, I set out for the second portion of my run, a nine mile whirlwind tour around the National Mall.

By the time I reached home, ragged from my 16 miles, Freddy's shift was over. The evening doorman, Andrew, returned my water bottle from behind the front desk. We exchanged half-hearted smiles, I thanked him, and went on my way, hobbling to the elevator.

To Andrew, and most of the world, I was just another anonymous runner. No one needed to know how far I'd run or what I was running for. Not even Freddy, my greatest marathon "frienemy" knew the circumstances under which I trained as a person with narcolepsy.

Two weeks later, on the day of my 18 mile run, I handed over my water bottle and sports energy packets to Freddy. He took my things and asked how far I would be going.

"Wow, 18 miles." He marveled in the moment, with a sparkle in his eye. "I can tell you are very determined."

"Well yes, I think I am."

"When you come back, I'm going to give you something special. I'm going to give you a new name – a Kenyan name!"

I smiled and left for my run with an extra pep in my step, looking forward to returning home to my new Kenyan name. I concentrated on my music and my walk breaks. The time passed fairly quickly.

After seven miles, I returned for my first hydration break. Freddy handed me my water and sports energy packet.

"Can I have my name now?"

Freddy laughed. "No, of course not. You're not done running yet. I'm leaving soon, so tomorrow – I'll give you your name."

Patience wasn't my best virtue. No matter, 11 miles stood between me and today's finish line. I headed out again to run Connecticut Ave – the steady incline toward the Maryland border was good practice for the Boston Marathon's Heartbreak Hill.

A few minutes into mile eight, just past the National Zoo, a sharp sensation cut under my right knee. I stopped short, startled. It was a familiar sensation but one I hadn't felt in years. My mind raced back to that fateful spring when I had first experienced this pain under my knees.

I reached down, touched my knees, and sighed with frustration.

A family walked toward me to enter the zoo, a little girl skipping ahead of her parents. I looked at her enviously. I wanted to be carefree too. Now, a dark cloud of anger and frustration hovered above.

I took a longer walk break – three minutes. The seconds moved slowly. The pain lessened as I walked, but when I picked up my pace, it returned.

Just keep going, I told myself. What else could I do? There was no choice. I stepped into the pain – 10 miles to go.

As time passed, a new sensation grew in my legs – a tightness in my quads. I tried stretching them out, but realized they were on the verge of cramping. I backed off. Still two to three miles from home, my mind raced ahead, picturing my body curled up in a cramped ball on the sidewalk.

I unzipped my jacket pocket to make sure I had my plastic bag of life-lines – three dollars wrapped around my driver's license and credit card.

It was getting late and the sun had ducked under thick clouds hours ago. The distance ahead was manageable only if my legs worked. The three dollars wouldn't get me far. I might need a cab but cabs didn't take credit cards here, and my roommate, Edward would still be at work.

My lifeline pack wasn't all that helpful. Despite visions of disaster, there was nothing else to do except keep running – cautiously, slower than ever, one foot in front of the other, hoping desperately that I'd somehow make it.

A wind whipped as I crossed a bridge and my body temperature dropped with my pace. There was no pleasure in this, trying to dodge ghosts of past failure and visions of future demise.

My arms and legs began shaking uncontrollably from the cold chill. With less than a mile to go, the forward motion of my body stopped on its own. My rock-like quads sat on daggered knees – a dysfunctional combination beyond my will power. I wanted nothing more than to finish this run. I needed the miles. I needed to report back to my blog followers that I was on my way to success. Above all, I was freezing and wanted nothing more than to be standing under a hot shower, or sitting still, or laying flat. My wet bra itched. Salty grime caked my cheeks – a mixture of sweat, wind and time.

I stood at a major intersection in Adams Morgan, wishing for a chair. The sidewalk never looked so comfortable. But also very cold.

Cars whizzed by. Pedestrians scurried into nearby stores and restaurants. Work hours were ending. Anonymous life moved around me, unaware of my broken body and collapsed spirit.

I hobbled slowly. It was less than a mile. A half hour later, I arrived back home, defeated. Andrew handed me my things from behind the desk. I didn't bother smiling, as I continued onto the elevator.

The next morning, I limped downstairs in loose-fitting grey sweat gear. Eighteen miles had done some serious damage to my body. It was too early for the mail, but I couldn't wait any longer. Freddy smiled when he saw me, knowing what I'd come for. He pulled out a Post-It note and wrote down one word – Wanjiru.

"This name means that you're a leader," he said.

I took the Post-It, thanked him and hobbled back upstairs.

Researching online, I found that Wanjiru was a traditional name among the Kikuyu people of Kenya. The Kikuyu represented 22 percent of the country's population. My name associated me with a clan known for leadership skills, strong warriors, and medicine men.

Another Kenyan runner shared my name, Samuel Wanjiru, who won the 2008 Olympics marathon, setting an Olympic record time of 2:06:32. In 2009, he won both the London and Chicago marathons, running the fastest marathon times ever recorded in the United Kingdom and United States, respectively.

After that, every time I walked in or out of the building, Freddy yelled out "Wanjiru!" from the front desk. I don't know if he knew my real name, but I liked this one better.

Once I recovered from my 18 mile run, I tried to continue running cautiously, but the pain under my knee worsened with each step. I went to a physical therapist right away, knowing that if there was any chance to make it to the marathon, professional help was needed.

I took the first available appointment with Matt, a physical therapist recommended by a friend. I described my symptoms and my history with tendonitis, and Matt moved my leg in various directions, testing my strength and flexibility. He asked me tons of questions – many I recognized from a few years ago. His deep concentration scared me.

Finally, he announced his prognosis. "I think you may be able to do it."

"Really?" My spine straightened with excitement.

"It's going to be a lot of work."

"Okay!"

"And we'll have to be cautious."

"Yes."

He led me through various stretches and strengthening exercises, then picked up a Styrofoam log. I'd seen these strange objects around gyms but had never used one. Matt taught me how to roll up and down the log in four different positions for about two to three minutes each, and when I found a problem spot on my legs, to lean on it for 10 seconds.

This seemed easy enough until I tried it. Problem spots ran up and down both legs. I breathed out heavily in eye-widening pain. The log was coming home with me, along with a long list of exercises and stretches.

Heavy drops of rain hit my nose as I left physical therapy. I hadn't brought an umbrella. Fifteen minutes never seemed so long, as I walked in the rain with a giant Styrofoam log tucked under my arm.

I should be running, not walking, I thought, shaking my head in disgust. I was supposed be overcoming narcolepsy, not *tendonitis*. I wanted to hurl the Styrofoam log into the gutter and sprint off to run 20 miles.

Running used to be simple. I went out, got sweaty and returned home – mission accomplished. There was no stretching, no strengthening, no icing, no sports energy packets, no medical bracelet, no fears, no protein-carb balanced diet. Now, running involved so many more factors. In a way, I was in a relationship with running and things just got complicated.

Regardless, I had to keep moving in the only direction I knew – forward. With only seven weeks to go, I was entering a new and unexpected phase of training – rehab. Matt outlined a plan that hopefully would restore the proper functioning of my knees so that my tendonitis wouldn't further impinge my training.

Finally arriving at my apartment building wet from the rain, I was happy to see Freddy at the front desk. He turned his head sideways to inspect the

Styrofoam log.

"It's a torture instrument meant to improve my running." I slouched over the marble countertop and explained that my knees weren't doing well. "It's all one big mess," I admitted.

He looked at me with steady strong eyes. "I can tell that you will complete this marathon."

For some reason, I believed him. He didn't seem to give out compliments or make predictions often.

"Thank you, but I don't know." And this was the truth.

"Yes, you will complete this marathon," Freddy reiterated. "You may not come in first place, but, second. You'll come in second. I've already predicted who will come in first!"

We broke out laughing together. I would have resisted, but his prediction that I would complete the marathon was more than enough. I'd be satisfied to come in second to a Kenyan.

The next weekend, I traveled to Boston for my sister Michelle's birthday. It was exciting to be back in my old stomping ground, if only for a quick trip.

I spent the afternoon wondering around the city with Michelle, finding almost everything exactly the same as when I'd left half a year ago. Yet, something was slightly different.

Walking down Boylston Street, I noticed a thick yellow line painted across the road, crossing Boylston right in front of the Boston Public Library, just outside Copley Square. Given the location, it occurred to me that *this* was the finish line of the Boston Marathon. I'd walked by this spot hundreds of times, but never noticed it.

A silly impulse surfaced. "I want to stand on the line," I told Michelle.

"Okay," she laughed.

"Will you take a picture of me?"

"You're insane."

"Please? For my blog?"

"Of course."

We waited for a break in the bustling traffic, and then I ran out into the middle of Boylston Street, turned around, opened my arms and tilted my head toward the sky. I wanted to know what it was like to stand here. Michelle took a few pictures and I scurried back to the sidewalk just as a taxi-driver began honking his horn at me.

On the line, arms open to a golden sunset, I could have cared less what anyone thought of me. I was proud to be attempting the marathon as a person with narcolepsy and eager to stretch my arms out there again in six weeks. Only then, I hoped to be greeted with more noise than the flimsy horn of one taxi.

I returned to DC, more determined than ever to continue my physical therapy routine and get myself across that line. On one of my first days back, I cleared the living room floor, plugged my marathon mega-mix into the stereo and dutifully began my stretch, strengthen, and roll routine.

After 30 minutes of stretching, I gladly moved on to strengthening exercises. I'd hated stretching until Matt introduced me to strengthening. My hips trembled uncontrollably as I performed the simple exercises. Now, I hated strengthening more than stretching.

After 20 minutes of pathetic shaky strengthening, I was thrilled to roll on to the foam log. On the last of my rolling exercises, a particularly strong problem spot surfaced, so I dutifully leaned into the tightness, huffing and puffing. The seconds on my stopwatch moved in slow motion. I tried to unfurrow my brow and think happy thoughts. *This is good for you, Julie.*

Intellectually, I knew the dull pain was tightness leaving my body, but that didn't make it hurt any less. I was nauseated and lost my ability to process these feelings with my usual even-keeled patience. Tears ran down my cheeks, a small stream attached to a sea of frustration.

I rearranged the furniture back to normalcy after I finished the final exercise. Over an hour had passed.

If running the marathon for myself, this would have been the end of the road. Narcolepsy was hard enough; I didn't need extra discomfort. Yet this race was much bigger than myself. Narcolepsy was more than just a cause to run for. It was the reason I ran, stretched, strengthened and rolled.

I was out of my comfort zone and didn't know what would happen. Nonetheless, running the marathon for narcolepsy was something worth fighting for.

With five weeks to go, Matt gave me the okay to try running again. The city was a bubble of sheer gloom, like a film noir, but my excitement to try running again propelled me outside. I set out for a modest 30 minute walk/run to the White House and back, rotating between 4 minutes walking and 4 minutes running.

A month earlier, I could have run 30 minutes in my sleep. With the flair of tendonitis in my knees, even this short distance was uncertain.

Sure enough, the knee pain surfaced within 20 minutes. This was a slight improvement but still disappointing after all my diligent work with Matt's exercises. I walked the rest of the way home in the ominous weather. Was I about to watch another nightmare come true?

NINETEEN
GOING THE EXTRA MILE

T HE PLANE DROPPED UNDER a thick layer of clouds, revealing the south side of Boston with little islands interspersed along the coastline. Land and sea washed into one another, like watercolor patches of green and blue paint. The miniature play-size buildings grew to life-size homes, garages, and cars.

I'd flown into Boston countless times – returning home, returning to school, returning to work, returning to my friends and family. Arriving on this day was different. My heart jumped and the intimidation set in.

Boston had never scared me before, especially not Marathon Monday, a festive state holiday when crowds of revelers took to the streets, the day the Red Sox played in the morning, the day some crazy 25,000 people ran from the burbs to Copley Square. For the first time, I felt like a visitor in my hometown, but I was still extremely proud of why I'd come to Boston.

At the baggage check, the first official sign welcomed the marathoners. Other passengers chatted about mile nine and Heartbreak Hill. I sized up my competition – skinny, athletic people.

My friend Elise greeted me with a big hug on the curb outside the airport. Traveling into the city together, we talked a mile a minute and I totally forgot why I was there, but not for long. When we arrived at her apartment, my home for the weekend, the marathon came back into focus in the best possible way. Elise had decorated bright pink and green posters with gobs of glitter to cheer me on for the marathon and taped them onto her guest bedroom door. A comforting warmth filled my stomach. All this for me?

After conducting a few news interviews downtown, I wandered around and took some photos. It was 40 degrees and lightly raining, but I barely noticed. I took my time, even posing in front of the Swan Boats for a photograph.

I visited the Boston Marathon Expo at the Hynes Convention Center to pick up my official bib and tracking device. When I handed my registration card to the volunteer, for some reason, I thought he hesitated, and I was ready to have a panic attack. What if there was a mistake and I wasn't really entered in the race? A second later, he passed me my official marathon pack and I felt like I'd won the lottery.

I went for my last training run in the rain around the Reservoir in Chestnut Hill. Usually, I would have complained about the weather, but I was so excited to be back running in Boston.

Although most of my training took place in Washington DC, this story truly began here, at Boston College Law School, a few hundred yards from Heartbreak Hill, where I'd fought a sleepiness of excruciating depths. It also began in my Fenway apartment and in the streets of Boston, where I collapsed to the ground with cataplexy and screamed in my car at night. I would never forget those difficult memories of adjusting to life with narcolepsy in Boston, but I was so excited to add a new and exciting chapter to this story.

Over the previous six months, I'd run over 312 miles toward my goal.

Now, I had only 26.2 more miles to go – a long way, but it was also the most exciting and straightforward part of the journey. I had nothing left to fear. I couldn't control my results – but I truly believed that every step I took was in the right direction.

The night before the race, my old roommate Tracy arranged for a group dinner at our favorite Italian restaurant in Fenway, down the street from our old apartment. Tracy and Natalie came from New York, Edward flew in from DC. Sophie brought a few more homemade posters to cheer me on. Most of our second year Halloween pageanteers attended the dinner, including Ms. Alaska, Ms. Nevada, Ms. Texas, and Ms. California, along with other friends from law school. We sat at a long table together, laughing, joking and most importantly, consuming copious amounts of carbohydrates. As a pasta-lover, I was in heaven.

"Are you excited?" Sophie asked.

I nodded.

"Are you nervous?" Tracy followed up.

I nodded stronger. I was both excited *and* nervous, but tried to deflect these inquiries by asking my friends about their jobs and their love lives. I didn't want to talk about the marathon, since a part of me was still in denial, trying to pretend that the race wasn't actually sneaking up on me so quickly.

After dinner, we said our goodbyes, took pictures, and hugged.

"See you at mile 13," Natalie said.

"See you at mile 22!" Edward added.

"See you at the after-party, Jules! You'll do great," Sophie hugged me last.

It was hard to say goodbye, but I had to get to bed to start my Xyrem doses. At this point, nothing stood between me and the marathon. No dinners, no conversations, no nothing. I was officially one night's sleep away from running 26.2 miles.

On the morning of the marathon, I awoke at 5:10 a.m., still a little groggy from my Xyrem. There was no time to waste. Out the door by 5:45 a.m., I walked from Elise's apartment down Chestnut Hill Avenue, with my neon yellow official marathon bag slung over my shoulder. This bag contained everything I needed for the long and momentous day ahead.

In Cleveland Circle, police and workers were busy setting up barricades. These barricades would be lined with marathon spectators in a few hours, including my friends. Although there was a serene silence to the early morning air, I could almost hear the chaotic cheers in the breeze. This small stretch of road was around mile 22 of the marathon route. I smiled to myself, thinking, *Next time I'm here, I will be four miles from finishing the Boston Marathon!*

I took the T train to the Boston Common, where the official marathon buses loaded marathoners to bring us to the start line in Hopkinton, Mass. I got in line to board a bus and made friends with the runners around me. Excitement was in the air. However, after an hour and a half of waiting in line, our enthusiasm wavered. When we boarded a bus at 8 a.m., I was physically shaking from the cold.

Okay, the worst is over, I thought. *We'll be in Hopkinton soon.*

Riding along the highway, I watched the trees, buildings and exits rush by. I couldn't believe I'd be running the *entire* way back. The long ride got even longer when our bus somehow ended up going the wrong direction for a bit. A simple trip to Hopkinton turned into a pilgrimage.

When our bus turned around to head in the correct direction, I realized that I needed a restroom. I'd dutifully hydrated all morning and now it was catching up to me. After an hour and fifteen minute bus ride, we finally passed a "Welcome to Hopkinton" sign around 9:15 a.m.

We must be close, I thought. *You can make it, Julie. Just hold tight.*

We were off the highway and on a small back road, when our bus came to a complete stop, stuck in marathon traffic. I shifted in my seat. A few other runners were getting off of buses in front of ours, and I assumed these brave souls were using the woods on the side of the road for the same reason I was sitting in pain.

A woman in the back of our bus yelled out, "We have a bathroom emergency! Are we allowed to get off?"

The driver shrugged ambivalently, so a young woman stood up and started toward the front of the bus. I stood up too.

"I'm coming with you!"

We examined the brush and soggy marsh-like area and tiptoed into a thicket of thorns, chatting about the race and how we should have used the Porta-Potties before getting on the bus. About 15 feet off the side of the road, with cars and buses passing by at a snail's pace, I took off my fleece and made an impromptu privacy shield for my new bathroom buddy. Then, she held it up for me. It was an all-time low – an act of true desperation – sad, comical, and sketchy all at the same time.

Back on the road, the traffic that had been stopped must have picked up considerably while we were in the thorny thicket with our pants down. Not only was our bus nowhere in sight, my official bag with all my gear, including my bib and tracking device, the two essential things needed to run the marathon, were gone with it.

My heart pounded. Would the woman sitting next to me on the bus grab my bag for me? And if so, how would I find her among the 25,000 other runners in the Athletes Village? My bathroom buddy, a bit smarter, had taken her bag with her off the bus.

We had no idea how far we were from the Village and the start line. We trekked along the side of the road, with cars passing by quickly now. Time passed by quickly, too. It was 9:45 a.m. Wave one of the marathon, my bathroom buddy's wave, started at 10 a.m. Wave two, my wave, started at 10:30 a.m.

Eventually, a man came running toward us, so we asked him how much farther to the Athletes Village. He looked at his watch.

"About a six minute run."

A six minute run? We were still three-quarters of a mile away, with little to no time before the start of the race.

We picked up our pace to a brisk run. My legs were stiff and uninterested in running and my lungs responded lethargically. I don't know what scared me more – the fact that I didn't have my bag or the fact that I was already out of breath. How would I run a marathon if I was already panting like a dog?

Eventually, the Athletes Village appeared up ahead. My bathroom buddy sped off to make her 10 a.m. start time. Miraculously, I saw the woman I'd been sitting next to on my bus, with *two* bags slung over her shoulder. I waved wildly and she waved back.

As she handed me my bag, I trembled with nerves and thanked her. When she left, I sat down on a curb to catch my breath. The marathon hadn't even started, and I'd already gone an extra mile, literally.

Once my nerves calmed down a bit, I pinned my official bib to my shirt and laced the tracking device into my left shoelace. On a patch of grass, I did some quick stretches. I'd expected to have hours to prepare. Now it was a matter of minutes. I gave up all hope of this marathon going well.

TWENTY
FLOATING

BY 10:30 A.M., I was tucked in between hundreds of other runners – a sea of people in front of me, and another sea behind me. Each individual was just a drop of water in a tidal wave of energy and excitement. At first, we stood still. Then we moved slowly. Walking turned to shuffling and shuffling became jogging. Crossing the official start line at 10:45 a.m., we were off and running.

The first half of the marathon, running through Hopkinton, Ashland, Framingham and Natick can be summed up in one snapshot – me being passed. Not a few runners, but every runner, passed me.

The gazelles flew by first, rubbing elbows with me as they whizzed by. Next, the young spunky runners, the smelly runners, the elderly runners, the limping runners, runners of all shapes and sizes, passed me. A man juggling while running backward passed me. Elvis passed me.

After seeing the wide variety of runners, every preconceived notion I ever had of what it takes to run a marathon was shattered. Seeing so many people with obvious limitations running around me was inspiring. Of course, it was also humbling to watch them pass me by, but I let them go and stuck to my plan. My own adversity wasn't as obvious on the outside, but still very real.

Running a marathon was one of the most personal tests of strength and endurance I'd experienced, yet taking this test among masses of other people, I had to remind myself over and over, that none of those other people mattered. I wasn't racing them, I was only racing myself. Since the beginning of my training, I'd had one and only one goal – to finish.

After my first 20 minutes of cautious running, I began my run/walk routine, as planned – running eight minutes and walking two minutes. The tendonitis in my left knee flared up in my sixth mile, which was exactly where Matt had predicted it. The knee pain became increasingly uncomfortable, but after each walk break, I started fresh and energized again, with little or no discomfort. It continued to bother me, but never became excruciating. The walk breaks saved me.

In the town of Wellesley, the all female Wellesley College students lined the barricades of the street, holding an extensive variety of "Kiss Me" signs. Everything from "Kiss me, I'm Alaskan" to "Kiss me, I'm a freshman." I didn't see them getting any kisses, and I can't imagine they actually wanted to kiss sweaty runners, but their signs were very entertaining. I looked down, away from the signs, to avoid any humorous thoughts from bringing on my cataplexy.

Also in Wellesley, was one of my cheering squads – Dad, Diana, Natalie, and her parents. I was worried that I might miss them, so when I spotted Dad's bright red Brown Squash Hat in the distance, I was filled with happiness. Dad waved and when I tried waving back, my knees weakened and I stumbled slightly but regained my footing without falling.

Dad hugged me tightly and we posed for a photograph together. My cheering squad said I looked great.

"Surprisingly, I feel great!"

"Are you sure?" Dad asked. "You stumbled – "

"Yeah, Dad. I'll be okay."

I didn't know if that was true. I didn't like feeling my cataplexy at mile 13, and was afraid that it might get worse, but there was very little I could do about it now. I had the emergency cataplexy medication in my fanny pack, just in case, but I really hoped to avoid taking it given the extreme nausea it caused me.

I continued on my way, passing the half way mark in 2 hours, 24 minutes and 55 seconds.

Wellesley was quickly followed by Newton, home to both Boston College Law School and Heartbreak Hill. I started to recognize the roads and landmarks around me. Miles passed where I only thought of logistics: *When is my next walk break? What song do I want to listen to next? When should I have my next sports energy packet? Gatorade or water?*

Keeping my gaze on the ground to avoid any further thoughts or emotions that might cause cataplexy, I was oblivious to most spectators. Still, I was aware of the generosity of adults and children, offering juicy slices of oranges, red Twizzlers, freeze pops, brownies and pretzels.

They held signs for individuals, for charity organizations, and even signs that said "Go Everyone!" There were homemade boards displaying the score of the Red Sox game, to keep the runners updated. People played cowbells and bongo drums, and others danced wildly on the balconies of houses and bars. If they had nothing else to offer, they held out their hands for high fives. It really was tremendous – not one inch of those 26.2 miles was without support.

I took my time going up the notorious Heartbreak Hill, running with short mini-steps. By then, I was no longer being passed, I was passing people. Reaching the top of Heartbreak Hill at Boston College's main campus, I thought of the nearby sleep lab where I'd spent the longest 24 hours of my life – chained to sleep. I began to let my legs go – stretching out to run as fast as they pleased. I stopped taking my walk breaks, surprisingly confident my body would hold up for the last few miles.

I sped down Commonwealth Avenue toward Chestnut Hill Avenue, knowing that a huge group of my friends were watching for me – the same place I had walked by at 5:45 a.m. I was happy to see them, and even happier not to feel any cataplexy in their presence. Their bright neon posters read "Flygirl: Go! Go! Go!" "Fly through that finish line. We love you, Julie!" "Go REM Runner" "Julie: this time you're the hero" and "Fly high, ZZZ's monster."

Edward high fived me. Elise snapped photos.

"You were booking it," Tracy said.

"Yeah, I feel great, actually. Thank you guys so much."

"Of course. We're so proud of you."

It was hard to leave them, but I had to keep going. In Cleveland Circle, my law school softball team captain and his girlfriend were waiting to run part of the way with me. We ran together through Washington Square, passing people left and right. At Coolidge Corner, I thanked them and continued on by myself toward Fenway Park and Kenmore Square.

When I saw the iconic red, white and blue Citgo Sign in Kenmore Square, it hit me full force – I would finish the Boston Marathon. My throat tensed, I was choking up, almost compulsively about to cry upon seeing the Citgo Sign. I held back from crying, not wanting the medical staff, who were watching us closely now, to think that I was in pain or that something was wrong.

Nothing was wrong – everything was so incredibly right, I was overwhelmed with emotion. Instead of crying, I smiled a big creepy gawking smile – totally bursting with happiness from ear to ear.

Rounding the corner of Boylston Street, I saw the finish line, just outside Copley Square. The blue and yellow marathon banners and international flags waived in the breeze. The crowds of spectators cheered loudly. It was a surreal image and hard to believe I was living it. I kept my gaze steady on the large banner over the finish line – the same finish line I'd been examining for months, the same finish line I'd photographed, wondering if I would cross it on marathon day and if I did, what would it feel like.

So what did it feel like as I raised my arms high in the air and crossed the finish line? It felt like floating, like being inside someone else's body – someone stronger and bolder – someone healthier than myself. To be honest, I never thought that this body would cross the finish line of the Boston Marathon, but I guess I proved myself wrong. In 4 hours, 41 minutes and 16 seconds, I finished.

Runner John Bingham once said, "The miracle isn't that I finished. The miracle is that I had the courage to start."

Looking back on this entire experience, I know that if it weren't for narcolepsy, I may never have taken on this challenge. My experience with narcolepsy, however difficult, awoke an urgency in me to live my life with intention. In my case, narcolepsy gave me the courage to start, and for that, I am forever grateful.

ACKNOWLEDGEMENTS

This dream would never have been realized without some very special people in my life. In particular, I would like to thank the following individuals:

To my father, Thomas John Flygare:

A year and a half after the Boston Marathon, on January 17th, 2012, my father lost his health battle to his heart. I can't describe this moment, other than to say that I always knew his heart would stop and mine would simultaneously feel torn out.

At the time, this book was two-thirds done. My dad had read early sections and quickly came around to supporting my writing efforts. While he never had the chance to read the full memoir, he lived this story with me firsthand.

If he were here today, I'd tell him that he was right – that my experience with narcolepsy *has* made for a greater life, something truly unimaginable on that dark December day when he made this prediction. Although narcolepsy continues to challenge me daily, I am coping well with diligent attention to my health, happiness, sleep and nap schedule.

As I continue working towards my dreams, my dad's love is still very much alive and a part of me. It's harder to see now, much like an invisible illness, there are some things we cannot see with our eyes, we must trust within our hearts.

To my mother: for fostering my creative spirit, athletic determination and passion for life. Thank you for believing in me and my writing potential. Your love and support has been invaluable in helping me to achieve my dreams.

To Aunt Julie: for cheering me on forever and always. I am so grateful for our shared life passions in the arts.

To my stepmom: for your positive spirit and strength. Thank you for loving Dad so unconditionally and openly embracing me and the narcolepsy community.

To my sister: for reading everything I've ever written and encouraging my progress. Your sisterhood support has meant so much to me.

To my brother: for your unconditional love.

To Gail Pean: for being the first person to read each chapter along the way. Thank you for the countless writing dates, warm meals and long discussions over tea and cappuccinos. Writing a memoir brought me to you - which has been a gift in and of itself.

To Alex Withrow: for being my grammar guru, editor and the love of my life. You generously gave your time and attention to help make my words fly. *I'm on my way. I'm on.*

To Professor Mary Ann Chirba: for believing in me before I dared to believe in myself. You gave me the courage to pursue this project and I'm quite certain none of this would have happened without you. Your mentorship changed the course of my life.

To Rebecca Rabin: for helping me navigate the emotional rollercoaster in the years following my diagnosis. Thank you for always listening with your heart.

To Dean W.: for understanding more about narcolepsy than I did at first and supporting me every step of the way.

To Lynn Stearns: for your excellent memoir writing class at the Bethesda Writing Center and your expert editorial work on the manuscript. You made this seem doable.

To Regina Ryan: for believing in my story despite tough odds.

To Sara Gorman: for your invaluable guidance on the publishing process and friendly support along the way.

To Ceci Sorochin: for your patience, kindness and creativity in designing the phenomenal cover and interior design. I wrote the words, you made them sparkle.

To Lucy Hillenbrand: for working with me to incorporate your breathtaking illustration into my cover design.

To Matt Spaulding: for your amazing photography.

To Dr. Emmanuel Mignot, Dr. Eveline Honig, Dr. Stephen Sheldon, Michelle King Robson, Mali Einen and Dr. Shelby Harris: for supporting my endeavor by reading my book and offering thoughtful kindhearted reviews.

To the Patterson family, the Carroll family, Melissa Buron, Lindsay Charles, Rachel Everett and Lynzey Kenworthy: for graciously reading pre-publication drafts of the book. You were my trust-worthy stepping-stones towards sharing this book with the world.

To Northside Social: for the delicious soy lattes that kept me awake to write this.

To my dear friends who have lifted my spirit along the way: Alexandra S., Amelia S., Ashley H., Carlyn B., the Cavnar family, Christine S., Dan H., David M., Emilee P., Freddy, Geraldine A., Jennifer W., Jess D., Julia G., Kerry E., Kristen L., Kristin J., Lianna O., Lillian R., Marcia C., Mee W., Neale M., Nicole N., Patricia H., Phoebe A., Stephen S., Rebecca M., Rebecca P., Sara K., Saraiah W., Sharon S., Sue D., Sze-Ping K., and Trinity H.

Last but not least, to the narcolepsy community: It never occurred to me that by me opening up, others would find strength and comfort in my words. Thank you for your messages of support that inspire me everyday.

Everyone's experience with narcolepsy is unique. While I've only told my own story here, I hope the voices of the 3 million people with narcolepsy worldwide come through between the lines, because this story really is about and for them.